**Tanja Petreska Ivanovska**
**Lidija Petrushevska-Tozi**
**Kristina Mladenovska**

**Probiotic and Synbiotic Food Products**

Tanja Petreska Ivanovska
Lidija Petrushevska-Tozi
Kristina Mladenovska

# Probiotic and Synbiotic Food Products

LAP LAMBERT Academic Publishing

**Impressum / Imprint**

Bibliografische Information der Deutschen Nationalbibliothek: Die Deutsche Nationalbibliothek verzeichnet diese Publikation in der Deutschen Nationalbibliografie; detaillierte bibliografische Daten sind im Internet über http://dnb.d-nb.de abrufbar.

Alle in diesem Buch genannten Marken und Produktnamen unterliegen warenzeichen-, marken- oder patentrechtlichem Schutz bzw. sind Warenzeichen oder eingetragene Warenzeichen der jeweiligen Inhaber. Die Wiedergabe von Marken, Produktnamen, Gebrauchsnamen, Handelsnamen, Warenbezeichnungen u.s.w. in diesem Werk berechtigt auch ohne besondere Kennzeichnung nicht zu der Annahme, dass solche Namen im Sinne der Warenzeichen- und Markenschutzgesetzgebung als frei zu betrachten wären und daher von jedermann benutzt werden dürften.

Bibliographic information published by the Deutsche Nationalbibliothek: The Deutsche Nationalbibliothek lists this publication in the Deutsche Nationalbibliografie; detailed bibliographic data are available in the Internet at http://dnb.d-nb.de.

Any brand names and product names mentioned in this book are subject to trademark, brand or patent protection and are trademarks or registered trademarks of their respective holders. The use of brand names, product names, common names, trade names, product descriptions etc. even without a particular marking in this work is in no way to be construed to mean that such names may be regarded as unrestricted in respect of trademark and brand protection legislation and could thus be used by anyone.

Coverbild / Cover image: www.ingimage.com

Verlag / Publisher:
LAP LAMBERT Academic Publishing
ist ein Imprint der / is a trademark of
OmniScriptum GmbH & Co. KG
Heinrich-Böcking-Str. 6-8, 66121 Saarbrücken, Deutschland / Germany
Email: info@lap-publishing.com

Herstellung: siehe letzte Seite /
Printed at: see last page
**ISBN: 978-3-659-71435-1**

TABLE OF CONTENTS

1.    **INTRODUCTION**................................................................3

      Probiotics..................................................................4

      Prebiotics..................................................................7

      Synbiotics..................................................................9

      Microencapsulation of probiotics............................................10

      Fruit juices as carriers for probiotics........ .................................15

2.    **AIM OF THE STUDY**.........................................................18

3.    **MATERIALS AND METHODS**.............................................20

3.1   Materials..................................................................20

3.2   Methods..................................................................20

3.2.1 Preparation of synbiotic microparticles......................................20

3.2.2 Experimental design in optimization of synbiotic microparticulated
      formulation.................................................................21

3.2.3 Characterization of synbiotic microparticles..................... ..................23

3.2.4 Stability assay of *L. casei* 01 during microencapsulation......................23

3.2.5 Viability assay of encapsulated *L. casei* 01.................................24

3.2.6 Swelling studies..........................................................24

3.2.7    Preparation of synbiotic carrot juice and evaluation of viable cell counts during fermentation and storage.......................................................................25

3.2.8    Chemical analysis of short chain organic acids.....................................26

4.       **RESULTS AND DISCUSSION**...........................................................27

4.1      Optimization of the formulation of synbiotic microparticles.................27

         Particle size distribution of the synbiotic microparticles.............................................................................29

         Surface charge of the synbiotic microparticles.......................................31

         Content of the cross-linking agent in the  synbiotic microparticles.............................................................................33

         Viability of *L. casei* 01 after preparation of synbiotic microparticles....34

         Viability of *L. casei* 01 in simulated gastrointestinal conditions............36

4.2      Physicochemical properties of the optimal formulation of synbiotic microparticles.............................................................................39

         Morphology of the synbiotic microparticles...........................................40

         Stability of *L. casei* 01 during microencapsulation...............................41

         Swelling studies....................................................................................42

4.3      Incorporation of free and encapsulated synbiotic in carrot juice.............43

         Survival of free and encapsulated *L. casei* 01 in carrot juice during fermentation and storage ........................................................................43

2

Survival of free and encapsulated *L. casei* 01 in non-fermented carrot juice ........................................................................................................46

Short chain organic acid profile of synbiotic carrot juice during fermentation and storage.........................................................................................................47

Short chain organic acid profile of non-fermented synbiotic carrot juice during storage.........................................................................................................50

5.    CONCLUSION.................................................................................................50

6.    ACKNOWLEDGMENTS.................................................................................51

7.    REFERENCE...................................................................................................52

## 1. INTRODUCTION

Food industry and especially dairy sector has been continuously revitalized through introduction of products characterized by their elevated nutritional value and pleasant taste, but also for the ability to exert positive effects on consumer's health (Casiraghi et al., 2007). Health benefits linked to consumption of food products can be strengthened by supplementing the conventional products with bioactive compounds and creating functional food products. Functional foods are foods providing additional benefits beyond the basic nutrition, as promotion of optimal health and reduction of risks for diseases (Roberfroid, 2002). Rapid development of functional foods in large extent is a consequence of modern living associated with economic growth and improved quality of life, which implicates various diseases related to the lifestyle. Fermented milk products, probiotics and prebiotics have gained increased interest for their potential impact on human health by regulating the gut microbiota composition and stability as support to host physiology (Ceapa et al., 2013). Among foods studied as carriers of probiotics, dairy matrix, either fermented or unfermented milks, is well documented. Dairy foods

3

are stored at refrigerated conditions and they are inherently related to probiotic bacteria providing suitable environment to support their growth and viability (Phillips et al., 2006). Hence, dairy products play important role in delivering probiotic bacteria to humans. Probiotic dairy products are recognized by the consumers as products that contain bioactive compounds beneficial for the general health and therefore easily accepted (Kiliç, 2013). Non-dairy products are also used as probiotic carriers, including fermented oat drinks (Klarin et al., 2008), cereal bars (Ouwehand et al., 2004) and juices (Gotteland et al., 2008). However, without significance of the carrier used, sensory profile of functional foods containing probiotics and/or prebiotics is still the most important marker of consumer's acceptance. Thus, development of functional dairy and non-dairy products have to consider several aspects such as functional properties of the product, sensory appeal, shelf-life, physicochemical stability, health claim approval and safety evaluation (Granato et al., 2010). On the other hand, it has been recommended that food enriched with probiotic bacteria should contain at least $10^6$ live microorganisms per g or ml at the expiry date in order to exert therapeutic effects (Manojlović et al., 2010). This level of viable probiotics, corresponding to the minimal level needed to obtain a clinical effect, is often quoted as $\geq 10^6$ cfu/ml viable cells in the small bowel and $\geq 10^8$ cfu/ml in the colon (Bertazzoni Minelli & Benini, 2008). Thus, developing a probiotic/synbiotic food product that contains relatively high level of active probiotic cells for providing positive health effects, while retaining physicochemical and sensory attributes, is a scientific and industrial challenge as well.

## PROBIOTICS

Probiotics are live microorganisms, which when administered in adequate amounts confer a health benefit on the host (FAO/WHO, 2001). Large range of microorganisms possesses probiotic properties, mainly bacteria, but also yeasts, such as *Saccharomyces cerevisiae* and *Saccharomyces boulardii*. Species belonging to the genera *Lactobacillus*,

*Bifidobacterium*, *Streptococcus*, *Enterococcus*, *Leuconostoc* and *Pediococcus*, which are normal constituents of the human gastrointestinal flora, are the most important probiotics. However, lactic acid bacteria, historically used for fermentation and preservation of food, are the most utilized probiotics in respect to safe administration (Ranadheera et al., 2010). Lactic acid bacteria and bifidobacteria are Gram-positive bacteria that live in a non-aerobic environment, but the growth of some *Lactobacillus* species can be supported in aerobic conditions (Anal & Singh, 2007).

It is well known that probiotic supplementation can alter the microbial balance to aid the host through several mechanisms, such as production of pathogen-inhibitory substances, competition with pathogenic bacteria for epithelial adhesion sites, nutrient competition and production, degradation of toxins and toxin receptors and modulation of immune and non-specific host responses (Prakash et al., 2011). The effects of probiotics are strain-specific (Luyer et al., 2005). Thus, when certain health benefit is claimed, it is very important to specify the genus and the species of the probiotic microorganism. Safety assurance of a new probiotic strain and probiotic products prior to introduction onto the market is required, characterized at a minimum with following tests according to the FAO/WHO guidelines (FAO/WHO, 2002): determination of resistance of the probiotic strain to antibiotics, assessment of metabolic properties of the strain (lactate production, bile salts deconjugation), monitoring of adverse effects in clinical studies, epidemiological studies of side effects incidence after approval for commercial use, identification of any substance secreted from the strain that may be toxic for mammals and determination of haemolytic potential of the strain (Petrushevska & Mladenovska, 2009). Further, all reported health effects are not sufficiently supported by the literature, thus for one probiotic strain to be used in humans, several characteristics have to be evaluated (Fig. 1). Clinical practice in respect to probiotic usage emerges screening of strains with high protective potential, profound studying of the mechanisms of action of a single strain or combinations and providing evidences from well-designed larger clinical studies to support the probiotic concept.

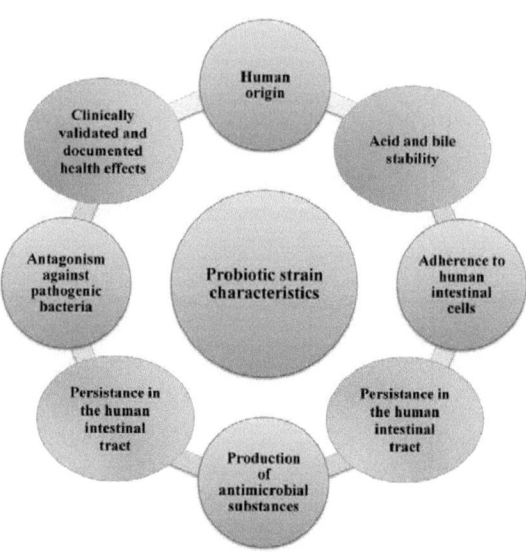

Figure 1. Selection criteria for a probiotic intended for human use

Potential implications of probiotics in prophylaxis and treatment of diseases within the gastrointestinal tract and beyond has been widely investigated. Therapeutic benefits include treatment of *Helicobacter pylori* infections (Gotteland et al., 2008) and antibiotic-associated diarrhea (Marteau et al., 2001), inflammatory bowel diseases (Huynh et al., 2009; Gentschew & Ferguson, 2012), irritable bowel syndrome (Almansa et al., 2012), allergic diseases such as eczema and atopic dermatitis (Kukkonen et al., 2007; Wickens et al., 2008) and gastrointestinal cancers (Orlando & Russo, 2012). Therefore, an important aspect of a probiotic is to remain viable during processing and

6

storage of food products and after administration in order to provide its health benefits. Exposure to light, pressure and high temperatures, presence of oxygen, moisture and salts are considered the main factors leading to significant loss of probiotic viability. After administration, passage of the probiotic through the low pH of the stomach and bile salts in the intestine may further reduce its viability. Prebiotic supplementation of probiotic products may potentially be useful for enhancing probiotic survival during processing (Corcoran et al., 2004). In addition, viability loss may be reduced by immobilization or microencapsulation of probiotic bacteria in a polymer matrix (Mitropoulou et al., 2013).

PREBIOTICS

Prebiotics have been defined as "non-digestible food ingredients that beneficially affect the host by selectively stimulating the growth and activity of one or a limited number of bacteria in the colon" (Gibson & Roberfroid, 1995). This definition was later reformulated as "prebiotic is a selectively fermented ingredient that allows specific changes, both in the composition and/or activity in the gastrointestinal microbiota that confers benefits upon host well-being and health" (Gibson et al., 2004; Macfarlane et al., 2006). Further, a successful prebiotic has to be safe, stable, resistant to digestion in the upper bowel and fermentable in the colon and able to promote the growth of beneficial bacteria in the gut (Gibson, 2004). Carbohydrates as oligofructose, fructo-oligosaccharides (FOS), inulin, galacto-oligosaccharides (GOS), transgalacto-oligosaccharides, soybean-oligosaccharides, gluco-oligosaccharides, xylo-oligosaccharides, gentio-oligosaccharides, isomalto-oligosaccharides, lactulose and polysaccharides as starch and pectins are considered to be effective prebiotics (de Vrese & Schrezenmeir, 2008). Most abundant prebiotics and their common sources are presented in Fig. 2.

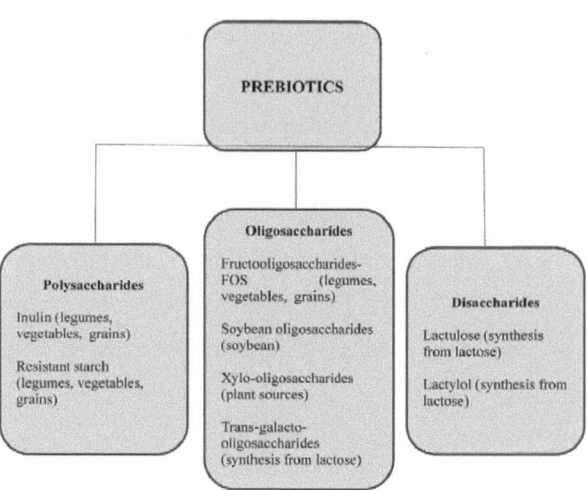

Figure 2. Classification of prebiotic compounds and sources

It has been reported that ingestion of prebiotics enhances the intestinal absorption of $Ca^{2+}$ and $Mg^{2+}$, beneficially affecting the bone mineralization and lipid metabolism as well preventing some types of cancer (Roberfroid, 2007b; Saad et al., 2013). Oligosaccharides have been found to serve as a source of energy for colonocytes, interfering with apoptosis, cell proliferation and differentiation (Duncan et al., 2002) and promote the growth of lactobacilli and bifidobacteria in the colon (Guarner, 2013). Majority of studies on prebiotics have focused on inulin-type fructans (inulin, FOS) and GOS as they have been linked to long-lasting and safe commercial use (Macfarlane et al., 2008). Oligosaccharides reaching the colon intact are fermented by colonic bacteria to short chain fatty acids (SCFAs) followed by production of gases (Roy et al., 2006; Meyer & Stasse-Wolthuis, 2009). These oligosaccharides are known as bifidogenic prebiotics (Birkett & Francis, 2010). Acetate, propionate and butyrate, as the main SCFAs, and lactate, as an important intermediate in the formation of SCFAs, are thought to be beneficial to host health. Namely, they have been found to alter gut integrity and to possess anti-inflammatory, antimicrobial and anti-carcinogenic effects, thus playing significant role in maintenance of gut and immune homeostasis. Among these, butyrate is preferred metabolic substrate of colonocytes and can stimulate various mucosal barrier functions (Tan et al., 2014).

SYNBIOTICS

Synbiotic refers to a synergism between probiotics and prebiotics. The presence of the prebiotic compound may improve the probiotic survival in food products and during transit in the upper part of the gastrointestinal tract, thus enhancing the probiotic effect in the colon. Several studies have reported a positive effect of the prebiotics added to dairy products, both on the viability of probiotic bacteria and on the physicochemical attributes (Castro et al., 2009a; Castro et al., 2009b; Oliveira et al., 2009; Oliveira et al., 2011a; Oliveira et al., 2011b; Debon et al., 2012). *Lactobacillus casei* (LC-1) has shown significantly higher viability during storage and in simulated gastrointestinal conditions when adhered to the oat bran, while a dairy fruit beverage obtained with the probiotic oat bran was well accepted by consumers (Guergoletto et al., 2010). Fresh-cut apple wedges with synbiotic properties and counts of probiotic bacteria comparable to commercially available dairy products (ca. $10^8$ cfu/g) have been developed using *L. rhamnosus* GG as probiotic and inulin and oligofructose as prebiotics (Rößle et al., 2010). Application of prebiotics as co-components for microencapsulation of probiotics or immobilization of probiotics in prebiotic edible films has also conferred a beneficial effect on cell viability (Fritzen-Freire et al., 2012; Soukoulis et al., 2014). From the clinical perspective, a randomized controlled trial investigating the benefit of probiotic, prebiotic and synbiotic treatment involving 100 patients with ulcerative colitis has indicated that the synbiotic therapy significantly increased the quality of life compared to the probiotic or prebiotic treatment alone (Fujimori et al., 2009).

Literature data suggest higher effectiveness of probiotics and prebiotics as a synbiotic combination. The subject of importance to obtain an effective synbiotic and to achieve an expected synergistic effect is to select a proper prebiotic substrate for a specific probiotic strain (Huebner et al., 2007).

MICROENCAPSULATION OF PROBIOTICS

Health benefits from the probiotics incorporated alone or as synbiotics into a range of food and pharmaceutical products are strongly dependent on their ability to survive and multiply in the host. A variety of approaches are utilized for enhancing probiotic viability compiling selection of bile and acid tolerant strains, stress adaptability, inclusion of oxygen scavengers, selection of appropriate packaging materials, two-stage fermentation and microencapsulation (Sarkar, 2010). Microencapsulation improves delivery of probiotics through enhanced stability (Champagne & Fustier, 2007), easier handling and storage of the cultures, with minimal influence on the sensory appeal (Picot & Lacroix, 2003b). This process forms continuous coating around an inner matrix that is wholly contained within the capsule wall as a core of protective material. The term immobilization can be interchangeably used, but refers to the enrobing of a material within or throughout a matrix (Mitropoulou et al., 2013). Microencapsulation/immobilization permits diffusion of molecules essential for cell metabolism, such as nutrients, oxygen and growth factors into the matrix, thereby supporting the viability of the cells and the outward diffusion of waste products (Talwalkar & Kailasapathy, 2004b; Mitropoulou et al., 2013). Hence, this approach for achieving improved viability of probiotic cells is advantageous compared to the others mentioned above. Microencapsulation could also enable controlled and targeted release, by depositing the entrapped cells across the small and large intestine (Cook et al., 2012). In order to enhance the probiotic viability during processing, storage and after administration, microencapsulation of probiotics using various techniques (e.g.

extrusion, emulsion, spray-drying, spray-coating, phase separation, coacervation and immobilization in fat and starch granules) may be utilized (Favaro-Trindade et al., 2011; Burgain et al., 2011; Cook et al., 2012). Literature data suggest usage of new technologies that do not involve severe conditions such as high temperature and solvents and allow production of highly desired smaller particle size. An example is usage of high-voltage spinning method known as electrospinning or electro-spraying technique to produce capsules in the micro, sub-micro and nano range through the action of an external electric field applied between two electrodes and imposed on a polymer solution or melt (Torres-Giner et al., 2010; López-Rubio et al., 2012). Electrospinning technique was successfully applied to encapsulate the probiotic *B. animalis* subsp. *lactis* in food hydrocolloids for functional food applications (López-Rubio et al., 2012). For preparation of probiotic sub-microcapsules, phospate-buffered saline and skimmed milk were utilized as media, while a carbohydrate pullulan and whey protein concentrate (WPC) as encapsulation materials. Electro-sprayed hydrocolloid-based structures showed protection ability and prolonged survival of the cells during storage at 4 °C and 20 °C and at various relative humidity (0, 11, 53 and 75%), with the WPC demonstrated better protection of bifidobacteria compared to pullulan. Other novel approach for food products is incorporation of probiotics into lipid microparticles due to the properties of the lipid matrix to block the exposure of probiotic cells to water and other stress agents like $H^+$ (Pedroso et al., 2012). Additional benefit of the lipid component is the easy digestion, favored by lipases in the intestine, which enables release of incorporated bacteria at the site of action (Favaro-Trindade et al., 2011). The technique of spray-chilling is similar to spray-drying method and is based on the injection of cold air which enables a molten matrix that contains the bioactive compound to solidify in the form of fine droplets (Champagne & Fustier, 2007). Spray-chilling may use lipids as wall materials and this was successfully applied in production of solid lipid microparticles using an interesterified fat with palm and palm kernel as a meltable carrier or

11

encapsulating agent (Pedroso et al., 2012). In this study, the viability of *B. lactis* in simulated gastric and intestinal fluids was not improved by microencapsulation since the cells both free and encapsulated have shown to be resistant, while in the same conditions, protection of *L. acidophilus* was provided. Spray-chilling method has the potential of scale-up for microencapsulation of probiotics since promising results in respect to the probiotic viability have been observed during refrigerated and frozen storage. In addition, morphology and size of the microparticles obtained by spray-chilling would not implicate the food texture. Further, alginate microbeads, 10-40 μm in size, encapsulating the probiotics *L. rhamnosus* GG and *L. acidophilus* NCFM have been developed by a novel technique involving dual aerosols of alginate solution and $CaCl_2$ cross-linking solution (Sohail et al., 2012). The survival of these two bacteria was not significantly enhanced by encapsulation. Namely, non-encapsulated *L. rhamnosus* GG cells were found to have excellent viability, while viability of both encapsulated and non-encapsulated *L. acidophilus* NCFM in orange juice, stored at 4 °C and 25 °C, was significantly reduced. In addition, encapsulation of *L. rhamnosus* GG significantly reduced acidification in the orange, peach and pear juice at both temperatures, showing the potential to reduce possible negative sensory effects caused by the probiotic itself in the fruit-based products. Microparticulated formulation containing *L. casei* 01 was developed using emulsion method followed by additional coating with whey proteins (Smilkov et al., 2014). Optimizing the combination of microencapsulating material using full-factorial design, the *L. casei*-loaded whey protein-Ca-alginate microparticles with favorable physicochemical, biopharmaceutical and biological properties have been prepared. The probiotic microparticles maintained the viability of *L. casei* 01 above the suggested therapeutic minimum after the manufacture and during exposure to simulated gastrointestinal conditions, indicating suitability to develop functional foods or pharmaceuticals. However, the spray-drying method for microencapsulation of the probiotic bacteria enables production of stable microparticles, with lower diameters and

12

more homogenous size distribution (Picot & Lacroix, 2004; Petrović et al., 2007; Menshutina et al., 2010). In addition, spray-drying is widely used due to its low cost, ability to process large volumes of solutions on a continuous basis, making the process easily adaptable to industrial applications (Kailasapathy et al., 2002; Mortazavian et al., 2007). Spray-drying method was applied to optimize the microencapsulation of *L. acidophilus* NRRL B-4495 and *L. rhamnosus* NRRL B-442 in raspberry juice to offer fruit powder with high probiotic viability (Anekella & Orsat, 2013). In this study, maltodextrin was used due to its prebiotic potential, but dextrose was shown to be a better carbon source to support the growth of the two probiotic strains. MRS medium acted as a better heating medium than raspberry juice during the sub-lethal heat shock pre-treatment. Based on the results, authors have concluded that the choice of the microencapsulating agent and the interactions among probiotics, carbohydrates and prebiotics are important to be studied to ensure better bioavailability. In addition, health benefits have to be evaluated in the presence of food matrix rather than isolated pure cultures.

Literature data summarize a spectrum of biopolymers that have been successfully utilized to provide safe transit of active probiotic cells through the upper GIT as coating materials (e.g. alginate, chitosan, gellan and xanthan gum, gelatin, pectin, κ-carrageenan, cellulose acetate phthalate, starch, milk proteins, whey protein gels) (Anal & Singh, 2007; Burgain et al., 2011; Mitropoulou et al., 2013). From the functionality point of view, encapsulating materials have to provide mild conditions for encapsulation, be biocompatible, non-toxic to the cells and host, impermeable for antibody-sized molecules, have sufficient membrane permeability and ability to overcome the acidic and enzymatic environment of the stomach and to increase adherence capacity and residence time of the probiotics in certain segments of the GIT as are the terminal ileum and colon. Because one material could not possess all these properties, usually, combinations of biocompatible materials with different properties are used. Combining the encapsulation materials may provide further benefit to the probiotic survival in unfavorable conditions. The study of Sohail et al., (2012) demonstrated that viability of probiotics in fruit juices is species dependent and microencapsulation in alginate beads only is not sufficient to protect sensitive probiotics from death. Hence, additional coating of alginate beads with materials like chitosan and poly-lysine may improve the stability of some probiotic species. Combination of chitosan and alginate for microencapsulation of bioactive molecules is frequently used due to the possibility for forming semi-permeable membrane between the positively charged chitosan and negatively charged alginate, which could not be dissolved in the presence of $Ca^{2+}$ chelators or anti-gelling agents (Chávarri et al., 2010; Petreska Ivanovska et al., 2012; Petreska Ivanovska et al., 2014a). Our recent comparative study of viability of the same probiotic strain *L. casei* 01 microencapsulated by emulsion using alginate and whey proteins and spray-drying method using alginate and chitosan indicated effective preservation during manufacture and storage at 4 °C in both cases (Petreska Ivanovska et al., 2014b). However, prolonged viability of *L. casei* 01 above the therapeutic level (> $10^6$ cfu/g) was assured for 6 months in whey protein-Ca-alginate microparticles and for 4 months in spray-dried chitosan-Ca-alginate microparticles, even with the prebiotic included in the second formulation. This observation may be owing to the more stressful conditions of the spray-drying process, but also to different properties of the encapsulating materials applied. Conjugates obtained between amino groups in proteins and the reducing-end carbonyl residues in saccharides, generally have superior surface stabilization properties, compare to their components before conjugation (Livney, 2010). The high protective potential of whey proteins in a view of probiotic viability is probably due to their buffering capacity which provides good shielding for encapsulated *L. casei* 01 against harsh conditions. The polyelectrolyte complex between alginate and chitosan, cross-linked with calcium ions, is relatively porous, while whey

14

proteins create strength anchorage for the cells that are embedded into the protein milieu (Doherty et al., 2010), thus the cells may retain their stability longer.

Although the coating of alginate beads with polycations and their functionality as drug carriers have been extensively studied, the search for optimal composition model for the encapsulating materials and method for microencapsulation of probiotics continues in order ability of the microparticulated systems to control and target the delivery of the probiotics to be improved and probiotic viability enhanced.

## FRUIT JUICES AS CARRIERS FOR PROBIOTICS

Fruit juices are interesting carriers for probiotics as they have pleasant taste profile and refreshing characteristics, inherently contain essential nutrients like vitamins and minerals, and are recognized as healthy and attractive for all age groups (Luckow & Delahunty, 2004; Sheehan et al., 2007; Gobbeti et al., 2010). Another cause for the favored development of non-dairy probiotic foods compared to dairy probiotic foods is the lack of dairy protein allergens, absence of cholesterol and lactose intolerance (Ray & Sivakumar, 2009; Granato et al., 2010). Moreover, there are no starter cultures in fruit juices like yoghurt which can compete with probiotics for growth factors and nutrients during storage, while certain antioxidants (ascorbic acid, poly phenols) are naturally present in fruit juices and can protect sensitive probiotic bacteria from oxygen due to the production of hydrogen peroxide (Sohail et al., 2012). Vegetable and fruit juices due to these advantageous properties are good candidates as probiotic vehicles (Soccol et al., 2010; Do Espírito Santo et al., 2011). However, in these matrices bacteria could need protection from the acid conditions because juices are generally too acidic to enable good probiotic stability during storage (Champagne et al., 2005). Favorable stability of probiotics in fruit juices can be reached by selection of strains that are less acid-sensitive and maintaining the pH of the product above 4.0 (Champagne & Gardner, 2008). The study of Nualkaekul & Charalampopoulos (2011), in which compositional design with model solutions and fruit juices were used to investigate the survival of *L. plantarum* NCIMB, has shown that presence of certain compounds like proteins and dietary fibers seem to protect the cells during storage (orange, blackcurrant, pineapple), while much lower cell survival than expected was found in pomegranate and cranberry juice. Since good cell survival in lemon juice with the lowest pH (pH~2.5) was observed, it was concluded that the presence of antimicrobial compounds, such as phenolic compounds, may contribute to fast reduction of cell viability in pomegranate and cranberry juice. In contrast to the results for the survival of *L. plantarum* in fruit juices during refrigerated storage for 6 weeks, the concentrations of citric acid, dietary fiber and total phenol did not affect the survival, while water activity and pH led to decreased viability during storage of reconstituted fruit juices (Nualkaekul et al., 2012). In this study, multiple regression analysis was applied to investigate the main factors influencing survival of *L. plantarum* in instant fruit powders produced by mixing together freeze-dried fruit powders and freeze-dried cells during long-term storage at room temperature and after reconstitution in fruit juices for up to 4 h. Results indicated that the instant juice powders are convenient carriers of probiotic cells and represent good alternatives to highly acidic fruit juices. Additional supplementation with inulin and gum arabic demonstrated considerable protective effect on the survival in the harshest conditions of cranberry juice, which was likely due to a physical interaction between the cells and the carbohydrates. Taking all factors into account, incorporation of probiotic microencapsulated systems is the most convenient for manufacture of functional food products at the same time improving the functional value of the product and ensuring protection of living cells from unfavorable conditions (Sohail et al., 2012). In addition, encapsulation technology may offer protection of viability loss after ingestion of the probiotics, especially during exposure to unfavorable acidic conditions in the upper gastrointestinal tract and antimicrobial effects of bile salts solutions (Sánchez et al., 2012).

Carrot juice is an interesting medium to prepare a functional product due to the presence of functional nutrients such as vitamins A, D, K, E, B, and C and minerals (sodium, potassium, calcium, ferrous, phosphorus) as well as carotenoids (β-carotene) which stimulate the synthesis of vitamin A. Different compounds with anti-oxidative properties which may have an important role as inhibitors of free radicals production and subsequent oxidative processes related to the onset of cardiovascular diseases or cancer, are also found in carrot juice (Krinsky et al., 2005). Some authors have even reported that the carrot juice containing *Bifidobacterium* strains (Kun et al., 2008) and cashew apple juice enriched with *Lactobacillus casei* (Pereira et al., 2011) allowed probiotic cells to grow, maintaining the viability of the probiotic at high level for determined time period. However, sensory off-flavors of these fruit juices were not well accepted (Luckow & Delahunty, 2004a), pointing to the factors that are challenging issues for the food industry. The most important is that probiotics must retain viability and the ability to confer a beneficial effect, but without detriment to the sensory properties of the food product and without compromising its safety (Sánchez et al., 2012).

Fruit and vegetable juices are seldom used as fermentable media for encapsulated cells. According to our knowledge, immobilized cells of *L. acidophilus* were used to ferment banana puree (Tsen et al., 2004) and tomato juice (King et al., 2007; Tsen et al., 2008) and it was observed that the number of viable cells during fermentation increased significantly compared to the free cells. The survival rate of several probiotics was comparatively evaluated in orange and apple juices, with better viability of encapsulated cells during 5-week storage (Ding & Shah, 2008). Nazzaro et al., (2009) investigated the ability of *L. acidophilus* encapsulated within an alginate-xanthan-inulin matrix to ferment carrot juice and to maintain viability in gastrointestinal conditions and during 8 weeks of cold storage. It was found that alginate matrix and synergy between the probiotic and prebiotic used protected the bacteria during storage in carrot juice,

17

incubation in gastric juice, and subsequent incubation in pancreatic juice. In the study of Chaikham et al., (2012), the influence of encapsulated probiotics *L. acidophilus* LA5 and *L. casei* 01 combined with pressurized longan juice on colon microflora and their metabolic activities during exposure to simulated dynamic gastrointestinal tract was evaluated. Both encapsulated probiotics combined with pressurized longan juice enabled significant increase of bifidobacteria and decrease of pathogenic bacteria in all colons, leading to significant formation of lactic, propionic and butyric acid and acetic acid to the lesser extent. These results indicate that encapsulation of probiotic cells and combination with juice rich in carbohydrates, fiber, minerals and other bioactive compounds (ascorbic, gallic and ellagic acid, total phenols) retains and supports the cells metabolic activities that are positively associated with beneficial health effects.

## 2. AIM OF THE STUDY

The development of non-dairy probiotic products is a part of the food industry activities towards utilization of abundant natural resources for production of high quality functional products (Granato et al., 2010). Despite the potential of juices for healthy products development, moderate research activity is applied in this field. While probiotic bacteria can be easily added to other cultures in dairy products, supplementation of juices with probiotics is more complex process. The main issue in the development of these products is maintenance of the probiotic viability during manufacture and storage as well as during passage through the gastrointestinal tract (Ying et al., 2010). Considering the properties that are required for a novel probiotic or synbiotic juice, comprising favorable sensory profile with improved health promoting effects, using microencapsulated probiotic/synbiotic may be an appropriate choice to prepare functional juice. In addition to the protective capacity of the coating materials, the *in situ* delivery of probiotic bacteria along the gastrointestinal tract may be enhanced by selecting materials with convenient biochemical properties (Chen et al., 2013).

18

Hydrophilic polymers like alginate and chitosan possess excellent mucoadhesive properties as their structures involve charged and/or non-ionic functional groups able to form hydrogen bonds with mucosal surfaces (Khutoryanskiy, 2011).

Considering the important aspects in the development of probiotic/synbiotic juice, the aims of the study included:

➢ Preparation of synbiotic (*L. casei* 01 and FOS) loaded chitosan-Ca-alginate microparticles. For this aim, spray-drying method was used to obtain synbiotic loaded Ca-alginate microparticles, which were subsequently cross-linked by $CaCl_2$ and coated with chitosan;

➢ Evaluation of the influence of the formulation factors i.e. concentrations of coating materials and cross-linking agent on the viability of the microencapsulated *L. casei* 01 during microencapsulation and gastrointestinal exposure. For this aim, set of experiments was designed and carried out using $2^3$ full factorial design. Response surface methodology (RSM) was used to determine the optimal ratio of the formulation factors in respect to the physicochemical and functional properties of the synbiotic microparticles;

➢ Microbiological determination of survival rate of *L. casei* 01 during microencapsulation by spray-drying and subsequent freeze-drying and stability of the encapsulated cells in simulated gastric and bile salts juices as well as cells release in the simulated colonic conditions to assess the therapeutic potential;

➢ Physicochemical characterization of the synbiotic loaded chitosan-Ca-alginate microparticles, comprising determination of particle size distribution, zeta potential, Ca-content, morphology and structure of the particles as well as possible interactions between the polymers, probiotic and prebiotic;

➢ Development of synbiotic juice with enhanced viability and metabolic activity of the probiotic *L. casei* 01 by adding the synbiotic microparticles to the carrot juice. Carrot juice was inoculated with non-encapsulated synbiotic (free *L. casei* 01 and

FOS) and synbiotic loaded microparticles to compare the survival rate of the probiotic and the production of lactic and acetic acid as *in vivo* promoters of probiotic's growth during fermentation and storage of the fermented and non-fermented beverages.

## 3. MATERIALS AND METHODS

### 3.1 Materials

As an encapsulating agent for manufacturing of synbiotic microparticles, sodium alginate (Protanal LF 10/60 LS, fG 35-45%), which was kindly donated by IMCD, FMC BioPolymer (Ayrshire, UK), was used. Chitosan with deacetylation degree $\geq 85\%$ and low viscosity 342 (viscosity of 10 mg/g solution in acetic acid 20-100 mPa s, $M_w$ 150 kDa) (France Chitine, Marseille, France) was used for coating of spray-dried microparticles, while the cross-linking procedure was performed with $CaCl_2$ (Merck, KGaA, Darmstadt, Germany) in previously prepared solution of chitosan and $CaCl_2$ in acetic acid (Merck, KGaA, Darmstadt, Germany). Freeze-dried probiotic culture of *Lactobacillus casei* 01 was purchased from Chr. Hansen, Hoersholm, Denmark. FOS was supplied from Sigma-Aldrich, St. Louis, USA. Bile salts (Ox bile dried pure) used for preparation of simulated intestinal juice, de Man Rogosa Sharpe (MRS) broth, MRS agar and peptone water were supplied from Merck, KGaA, Darmstadt, Germany. All the reagents were of analytical grade.

### 3.2 Methods

#### 3.2.1 Preparation of synbiotic microparticles

Synbiotic microparticles were prepared by spray-drying method and further stabilized by freeze-drying (Petreska Ivanovska et al., 2012a). Shortly, freeze-dried probiotic culture *L. casei* 01 was inoculated into 5 ml MRS broth and incubated at 37 °C for 24 h under aerobic conditions. The cells were harvested by centrifugation at 1500 x $g$

20

for 10 min and washed with sterile peptone solution (1 g/L). An aqueous suspension of *L. casei* 01 with a cell load *ca.* 12 log cfu/g, FOS (1.5% w/w) and alginate was infused into a spray-dryer (Büchi Mini Spray Dryer B-290, Flawil, Switzerland) to obtain microparticles. The conditions of the spray-drying process were: nozzle diameter 0.7 mm, aspirator pressure 90%, atomizer pressure 600 Nlh$^{-1}$, flow rate 6 ml/min, inlet temperature 120 °C and outlet temperature 60 °C. Spray-dried microparticles were collected in sterile containers and then slowly added into previously prepared solution of CaCl$_2$ and chitosan in 1% v/v acetic acid under continuous stirring using a magnetic stirrer for at least 3 h at room temperature. The hardened microparticles were separated by centrifugation at 1500 x *g* for 10 min, washed with sterile saline solution and frozen at -20 °C. Afterwards, the microparticles were freeze-dried at 0.070 mbar and -50 °C for 24 h (FreeZone Freeze Dry System, Labconco, Kansas City, USA).

3.2.2 Experimental design in optimization of synbiotic microparticulated formulation

In order to obtain the optimal formulation of synbiotic microparticles, $2^3$ full factorial design was used to create a set of experiments. Two levels for the factors were defined, upper ("+") and lower ("-") level, and a zero level (center), in which all variables are fixed at their mean value, was also included in order to minimize the risk of missing non-linear relationships. However, the zero level experiment was not included in the calculation of the coefficients. Screening experiments were carried out with three independent variables that affect the experimental responses, sodium alginate in concentration limits of 1 and 4% w/w ($x_1$), chitosan in concentration limits of 0.1 and 0.5% w/w ($x_2$) and CaCl$_2$ in concentration limits of 0.5 and 5% w/w ($x_3$) (Table 1). All modeling analyses were performed using experimental design software program MODDE 8.0 (Software for design of experiments and optimization, Umetrics, Umea, Sweden). Regression analysis was performed on the basis of experimental results to

21

construct mathematical models. The coefficients of the model were obtained using response surface methodology to fit the experimental data to polynomial equation and to define the optimal formulation.

Table 1. *Experimental matrix for the series of synbiotic microparticles with L. casei 01 enriched with FOS; independent factors and experimental responses*

| Exp. no. | Independent factors | | | Viability of encapsulated *L. casei* (log cfu/g) | | | | Physicochemical properties | | |
|---|---|---|---|---|---|---|---|---|---|---|
| | $X_1$ Alginate (%, w/w) | $X_2$ Chitosan (%, w/w) | $X_3$ CaCl$_2$ (%, w/w) | Viability after freeze-drying | Viability in simulated gastric juice after 3 h | Viability in simulated intestinal juice after 6 h | Viability in simulated colon conditions after 24 h | Particle size $d_{50}$ (μm) | Zeta potential (mV) | Ca$^{2+}$ content (mg / 10 mg particles) |
| 1 | 1 | 0.1 | 0.5 | 7.26 | 4.32 | 2.27 | 0 | 8.74 | -20.8 | 0.43 |
| 2 | 4 | 0.1 | 0.5 | 9.67 | 7.15 | 4.49 | 3.89 | 9.22 | -21.71 | 0.49 |
| 3 | 1 | 0.5 | 0.5 | 7.94 | 6.06 | 4.94 | 4.81 | 6.70 | 25.42 | 0.51 |
| 4 | 4 | 0.5 | 0.5 | 8.60 | 6.50 | 4.82 | 4.18 | 12.47 | 24.6 | 0.35 |
| 5 | 1 | 0.1 | 5 | 10.73 | 7.85 | 7.01 | 7.06 | 6.86 | -18.54 | 1.01 |
| 6 | 4 | 0.1 | 5 | 10.79 | 8.66 | 7.22 | 7.14 | 6.68 | -8.86 | 1.07 |
| 7 | 1 | 0.5 | 5 | 10.24 | 8.49 | 6.64 | 6.69 | 6.68 | 16.81 | 1.22 |
| 8 | 4 | 0.5 | 5 | 11.30 | 9.62 | 8.46 | 7.67 | 8.77 | 21.56 | 0.94 |
| 9 | 2.5 | 0.3 | 2.75 | 10.98 | 8.64 | 8.04 | 8.31 | 8.26 | 13.90 | 0.88 |
| 10 | 2.5 | 0.3 | 2.75 | 10.90 | 8.66 | 8.07 | 8.26 | 8.29 | 15.10 | 0.84 |
| 11 | 2.5 | 0.3 | 2.75 | 10.96 | 8.75 | 8.02 | 8.24 | 8.18 | 15.00 | 0.87 |

An applied linear mathematical model to measure the response of the investigated factors was:

$$y = b_0 + b_1 x_1 + b_2 x_2 + b_3 x_3 + b_{12} x_1 x_2 + b_{13} x_1 x_3 + b_{23} x_2 x_3$$

where y presents the estimated response, $b_o$ is intercept of the linear model showing the average experimental response, coefficients $b_1$, $b_2$, and $b_3$ are the estimated experimental responses of the factors showing the main effects, while the coefficients $b_{12}$, $b_{13}$, and $b_{23}$ are showing two-factor interactions. The response surface plots illustrate the relationship between the factors and the responses by holding constant one of the three independent factors.

### 3.2.3 Characterization of synbiotic microparticles

The comparison in morphology of the mechanically untreated and grounded particles, both coated with chromium, was performed using high vacuum SEM technique (Leo 1450 VP, Oberkochen, Germany) at an accelerating voltage of 30 kV. Size distribution of the chitosan-Ca-alginate microparticles was measured by laser light scattering (Mastersizer Hydro 2000G, Malvern Instruments Ltd., Worcestershire, UK) and the mean particle size was expressed as $d_{50}$. The zeta potential of the suspended microparticles in 0.1 mM phosphate buffer (pH 6.8) was recorded using Zeta-sizer Nano ZS (Malvern Instruments Ltd., Worcestershire, UK). The calcium content of the microparticles was determined by atomic emission spectroscopy-inductively coupled plasma, AES-ICP (Varian, Palo Alto, USA) after degradation of the microparticles with $HNO_3$ (2.5 mg/ml) (Mladenovska et al., 2007a; Petreska Ivanovska et al., 2012a).

### 3.2.4 Stability assay of *L. casei* 01 during microencapsulation

Fourier transform infrared spectroscopy (FTIR) was used to determine the stability of the probiotic *L. casei* 01 during microencapsulation. FTIR-ATR spectra were recorded at room temperature using a Zinc Selenide crystal and Golden Gate[TM] ATR attachment (Perkin Elmer System 2000 FTIR, ATR-IR Golden Gate, Waltham, USA), in frequency range of 4000-400 cm$^{-1}$. In order to determine the possible molecular changes of the probiotic structure during the microencapsulation process, the spectra of non-encapsulated *L. casei* 01 and released from the microparticles were compared.

3.2.5 Viability assay of encapsulated *L. casei* 01

Viability of the encapsulated *L. casei* 01 cells was determined using plate-count method. Namely, the microparticles were dispersed in phosphate buffer solution (pH 6.9) until complete release of the probiotic cells. Then, *L. casei* 01 was plated in triplicate on selective MRS agar, incubated at 37 °C under aerobic conditions for 72 h and enumerated. The average of the results was expressed as colony-forming units per gram of sample (cfu/g). For viability tests in simulated gastrointestinal juices, method of Mokarram et al., (2009) was used, with slight modifications of the simulated gastric juice as Gbassi & Vandamme (2012) suggested presence of enzyme in its composition. Namely, the microparticles were incubated in simulated gastric juice (0.08 M HCl with 2 g/L NaCl and 3 g/L pepsin, pH 1.5) using a shaking water bath at 75 strikes/min (Haake, SWB 25, Burlandingen, Germany) for 3 h and in bile salts solution (0.05 M KH$_2$PO$_4$; pH 6.8 with 10 g/L filter sterilized bile salts) for additional 3 h. Washed microparticles were transferred in simulated colon medium (0.1 M KH$_2$PO$_4$; pH 7.4) (Mandal et al., 2006) and incubated up to 24 h.

3.2.6 Swelling studies

Swelling properties of the optimal formulation of microparticles were evaluated by measurement of the particle size in simulated gastrointestinal fluids with different pH values. Given amount of microparticles (30-40 mg) was suspended in 5 ml of acetate buffer (pH 1.5) and phosphate buffer solutions with pH 6.8 and 7.4, respectively. An exchange method was used to carry out the swelling test during stirring by magnetic stirrer at 300 rpm and temperature of 37 °C. At determined time intervals, the samples were removed from the swelling medium and assayed for particle size by Mastersizer (Hydro 2000G, Malvern Instruments Ltd., Worcestershire, UK). Percent swelling value was calculated according to the following equation:

$$[(D_t - D_0)/D_0] \times 100$$

where, $D_t$ and $D_0$ are the mean volume diameters of the microparticles at time t and in the dry state, respectively (El-Gibaly, 2002).

3.2.7 Preparation of synbiotic carrot juice and evaluation of viable cell counts during fermentation and storage

Carrot juice was prepared by extraction of washed and peeled carrots purchased at the local supermarket, with no added water, preservatives or any other nutrient. Then, the juice was pasteurized at 80 °C for 20 min. The initial cell concentration of 7.4±0.1 log cfu/ml was applied to ferment the carrot juice using *L. casei* 01 and FOS or synbiotic microparticles. This concentration was chosen according to the recommendations for minimum counts of 7.0 log cfu per g or ml of probiotic food to exert beneficial effects (Vinderola & Reinheimer, 2000). One sample of the carrot juice inoculated with free cells and one sample containing microparticles were firstly submitted to fermentation at 37 °C for 24 h and then stored at 4 °C. The cell population of non-fermented samples with free and encapsulated *L. casei* 01 was adjusted to 10.5±0.2 log cfu/ml. Another two samples were inoculated with free cells of *L. casei* 01 or *L. casei* 01 loaded microparticles, respectively, and then stored in refrigerated conditions for 6 weeks. In the juices containing non-encapsulated *L. casei* 01, the prebiotic FOS was added simultaneously with the probiotic cells. All samples of synbiotic carrot juices were packed into sterile Erlenmeyer flasks closed with cotton plugs.

The viability of *L. casei* 01 in all experiments was determined periodically during 24 h fermentation and then on a weekly basis for 6 weeks of storage. When enumeration of bacteria was performed, 1 ml of the sample was mixed with 9.0 ml of peptone water, vortexes for 15 s, then serially diluted with peptone water and the viable count was determined as it was described in a previous section. The same procedure was performed for samples with added microparticles, after removing the particles from the juice by filtration (Sandoval-Castilla et al., 2010). Viability assay for non-fermented samples was performed at the preparation step and then once a week during cold storage. The pH of synbiotic carrot juice was also examined simultaneously with the viability assays (pH meter PB-11 Sartorius, Goettingen, Germany).

3.2.8 Chemical analysis of short chain organic acids

The amount of short chain organic acids was determined temporary during fermentation and then once a week in a storage conditions by high-performance liquid chromatography using a HPLC system apparatus equipped with an ultraviolet detector (Agilent Technologies 1200, Palo Alto, USA). The method used by Wang et al., (2003) for determination of acid content in fermented soymilk was applied. Shortly, to determine the concentrations of lactic and acetic acid, 2 ml of 0.5 M $H_2SO_4$ were added to a 2-ml aliquot of the sample, thoroughly mixed for 30 s and centrifuged (12 000 x $g$ for 15 min). The obtained supernatants were filtered through 0.45 μm membrane (Minisart RC 25, Sartorius Stedim Biotech, GmbH, Goettingen, Germany). Samples were loaded onto a thermostatically controlled reverse phase column (250 mm x 4.6 mm, 5 μm, Discovery HS C 18, Supelco Park, Bellefonte, PA, USA) set at 40 °C and eluted with 0.005 M $H_2SO_4$ at flow rate of 1 ml/min. According to the method applied, a detection wavelength was 210 nm, while identification of lactic and acetic acids was done using their respective standards.

## 4. RESULTS AND DISCUSSION

*Lactobacillus casei* is an acid sensitive, rod-shaped, facultative heterofermentative lactic acid bacterium that can be isolated from a variety of environments including raw and fermented milk and meat or plant products, as well as the oral, intestinal, and reproductive tracts of humans and animals. It is a beneficial microorganism that helps to promote other beneficial bacteria and prevents the overgrowth of pathogenic bacteria in the human body. It has been reported that it can improve and intensify digestion, control diarrhea, reduce inflammations of the gut, reduce lactose intolerance and alleviate the symptoms of constipation, all leading to better function of the immune system (Marteau et al., 2002; Gill & Prasad, 2008). Recently, there has been intensive use of this probiotic in functional food products. However, many reports indicate poor survival of the probiotic in these products and also the survival in the human gastrointestinal system is questionable (Vidhyalakshmi et al., 2009). In our studies, 3-hour exposition to simulated gastric acid at 37 °C using a horizontal shaking water bath with 75 strikes/min (0.08 M HCl; 2 g/L NaCl; 3 g/L pepsin; pH 1.5) resulted in poor survival of *L. casei* 01, $2.68 \pm 0.28$ log cfu/g *vs.* $10.51 \pm 0.58$ log cfu/g as initial cell count, while with 10-hour continuous exposition to bile salts in pH 6.8 (0.05 M $KH_2PO_4$; 10 g/L bile salts), the viability of the probiotic decreased to $4.18 \pm 0.13$ log cfu/g. Considering that, providing *L. casei* 01 with a physical barrier against adverse environmental conditions could significantly improve its stability, thus ensuring its health effects.

### 4.1 Optimization of the formulation of synbiotic microparticles

With reference to the aim of this study, to obtain synbiotic juice with high probiotic viability using microparticulated carriers, the choice of the polymers was limited to food-grade materials. Our previous investigations (Petreska Ivanovska et al., 2012a) have suggested that the chitosan-Ca-alginate system is convenient to preserve viability of the probiotic *L. casei* 01 during spray-drying and in simulated gastrointestinal

27

conditions. Therefore, the concentrations of the formulation factors were optimized to obtain synbiotic microparticles with enhanced viability of *L. casei* 01 and adequate release profile in different regions of the GIT that were further used to prepare synbiotic carrot juice. In the preliminary investigations, in which the concentrations of the encapsulation materials, cross-linking agent, FOS and initial cell count were varied as well as the processing variables, it was found that the concentrations of encapsulating materials, alginate and chitosan, and of the cross-linking agent were the most significant factors affecting the physicochemical properties of the microparticles and viability of *L. casei* 01 during preparation and in simulated gastrointestinal conditions. Although several responses were monitored to select the optimal values of the formulation factors, the main concern was given to the viability of *L. casei* 01 in simulated gastric juice. This implication is accounted on the fact that the probiotics must first survive the deleterious effect of the gastric pH in order to reach the intestine where the bioadhesive properties of the delivery system are among the key factors for achieving prolonged residence time and effective colonization of the probiotic. The primary response, viability of the encapsulated *L. casei* 01 in simulated gastric conditions, pointed to the formulation factor with the lowest influence i.e. chitosan. In this respect and in conjunction with the other experimental responses as well, it was concluded that the optimal formulation of synbiotic chitosan-Ca-alginate microparticles should be prepared of 4% w/w alginate, 0.5% w/w chitosan and 5% w/w $CaCl_2$. This suggestion was deduced on the basis of narrow concentration range of chitosan (0.4-0.5% w/w) needed to produce microparticles with favorable zeta potential i.e. mucoadhesive properties, minimal concentration of 4.64% w/w for $CaCl_2$ to protect the probiotic cells in the acidic environment of the gastric juice and increased viability of the probiotic during microencapsulation, freeze-drying and in simulated gastric and intestinal juices with higher alginate concentration. Namely, when chitosan in concentration of 0.1% w/w was applied, negative values for the zeta potential of the microparticles were obtained (Table

1), which might lead to repulsive interaction with the negatively charged mucus glycoprotein. Therefore, a compromise was imperative and it was assumed that with decreasing chitosan concentration below 0.4% w/w, the viability of *L. casei* 01 in simulated gastric conditions would not be affected, but the surface characteristics of the microparticles would lead to decreased potential for interaction with the mucus glycoprotein. The high $CaCl_2$ concentration as a dominant factor in providing probiotic viability during preparation of synbiotic microparticles and their exposure to simulated gastrointestinal conditions is required for efficient cross-linking of microparticles i.e. mechanical stability of the microparticles. On the other hand, $CaCl_2$ concentration showed no significant influence on the zeta potential of the microparticles. In addition, positive values for zeta potential were obtained within the experimental range of alginate (1-4% w/w), pointing to no significant influence of the alginate concentration on this response. The experimental responses obtained for particle size and Ca-content of the microparticles was also monitored to confirm the favorable physicochemical properties of the optimized formulation.

Particle size distribution of the synbiotic microparticles

Particle size is an important factor affecting the survival rate and colonization of encapsulated probiotics, sensory properties of the probiotic food products and quality and stability of the pharmaceutical products. Depending on the method of microencapsulation, the size of the produced microparticles ranges in wide interval, usually from 5 μm to 3 mm. The large particles can negatively affect the textural and sensorial properties of the food products in which they are added (Sandoval-Castilla et al., 2010; Burgain et al., 2011). According to Truelstrup Hansen et al., (2002), particles with size below 100 μm are suitable for direct addition in numerous food products, but did not significantly protect the encapsulated bifidobacteria in simulated gastric conditions comparing to the free cells. However, small and controlled size particles are

29

more convenient for incorporation into food products due to the easier managing and higher stability (Cui et al., 2001). Furthermore, smaller particles are better for achieving successful adhesion and colonization in the gut, while large particles move faster through the colon and come rapidly in the descending colon prior defecation (Washington et al., 2001). In this study, the response for particle size was analyzed in conjunction with the minimal value required for successful encapsulation of the probiotic cells, usually 1 to 4 μm (Burgain et al., 2011), and the recommendation for particle size below 10 μm in order most foods to keep mouthfeel characteristics (O'Riordan et al., 2001). The method of spray-drying used in our study allowed production of stable microparticles, with mean volume diameter ranging from 6.7 to 12.5 μm within all experimental series (Table 1).

Table 2. *Regression coefficients of the experimental model*

| Experimental response | Regression coefficients | | | | | | |
|---|---|---|---|---|---|---|---|
| | $b_0$ | $b_1$ | $b_2$ | $b_3$ | $b_{12}$ | $b_{13}$ | $b_{23}$ |
| Viability of *L. casei* after freeze-drying | 9.834 | 0.599 | -0.121 | 1.274 | -0.019 | -0.319 | 0.126 |
| Viability of *L. casei* (pH 1.5, 3h) | 7.695 | 0.651 | 0.336 | 1.323 | -0.258 | -0.166 | 0.064 |
| Viability of *L. casei* (pH 6.8, 6h) | 6.240 | 0.499 | 0.466 | 1.619 | -0.074 | -0.026 | -0.284 |
| Viability of *L. casei* (pH 7.4, 10h) | 5.353 | 0.431 | 0.711 | 1.926 | -0.426 | -0.196 | -0.591 |
| Viability of *L. casei* (pH 7.4, 24h) | 5.781 | 0.540 | 0.658 | 1.960 | -0.453 | -0.275 | -0.618 |
| Zeta potential of microparticles | 4.748 | 1.588 | 19.788 | 0.433 | -0.605 | 2.020 | -3.345 |
| Ca content in the particles | 0.774 | -0.040 | 0.003 | 0.308 | -0.070 | -0.015 | 0.018 |
| Particle size | 8.267 | 1.021 | 0.389 | -1.017 | 0.944 | -0.544 | 0.086 |

Considering the values of the regression coefficients (Table 2), it can be concluded that the most significant effect on the particle size had alginate concentration ($x_1$), than

CaCl$_2$ concentration ($x_3$) and afterwards, chitosan concentration ($x_2$). With increasing alginate concentration, particle size increases and it decreases with increasing CaCl$_2$ concentration. In our experimental system, the particle size was optimized in respect to minimal CaCl$_2$ and chitosan concentrations required to achieve increased probiotic viability and favorable interaction of the particles with the intestinal mucosa, 4.64 and 0.4% w/w, respectively. Therefore, the minimal particle size that fulfils the mentioned criteria was the value of 8.19 μm (Table 1).

Surface charge of the synbiotic microparticles

Another factor that implies adherence property of the particles to the epithelial support of the intestine is the particle charge. There are literature data showing that probiotic cells are in general negatively charged (Pelletier et al., 1997). Our measurements of the zeta potential at pH 6.8 pointed that free cells of the probiotic *L. casei* 01 were also negatively charged (-16.4±0.7 mV). Various polymers are able to interact with mucus and may improve the residence time of the microparticulated delivery systems (Pliszczak et al., 2011). Mucoadhesive properties of hydrophilic polymers like alginate and chitosan are mainly due to forming of hydrogen bonds between charged functional groups and mucosal surfaces (Khutoryanskiy, 2011). The concentration of positively charged carrier, chitosan, was optimized to provide favorable interaction with the negatively charged glycoprotein from the mucus, to increase the mucoadhesion capacity and thus, to prolong the residence time of the encapsulated probiotic cells in the lower intestine. With measurements of the zeta potential for the series of microparticles generated with the experimental design, values ranging from -21.71 to 25.42 mV were obtained (Table 1). The values of the regression coefficients, $b_1$, $b_2$ and $b_3$ (Table 2) indicate that the surface charge of the synbiotic microparticles is dominantly affected by the chitosan concentration ($x_2$), while the effects of the alginate ($x_1$) and CaCl$_2$ concentration ($x_3$) are significantly lower, with the lowest influence of the

31

concentration of $CaCl_2$. The contour diagrams at Fig. 3 present the zeta potential values as a function of alginate $(x_1)$ and chitosan concentration $(x_2)$, while the $CaCl_2$ concentration $(x_3)$ is kept constant at 0.5% w/w (Fig. 3a), 2.75% w/w (Fig. 3b) and 5% w/w (Fig. 3c). Although, the best response for zeta potential of 26.3 mV at $CaCl_2$ concentration of 0.5% w/w was obtained, high $CaCl_2$ concentration was used due to its effect on the primary response i.e. viability of the probiotic cells in the acidic gastric conditions. At the optimum point for viability in simulated gastric medium (Fig. 3c), the zeta potential was predicted to be at least 14.3 mV, which satisfies the postulated surface properties of the prepared particles.

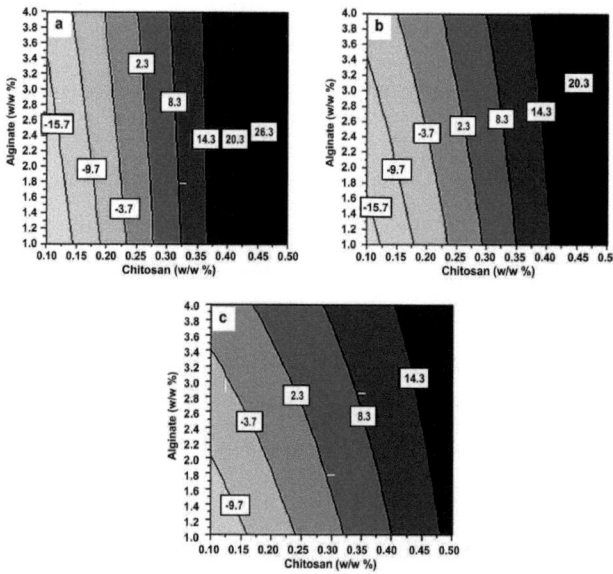

Figure 3. A contour diagrams for zeta potential of the microparticles as a function of alginate and chitosan concentrations at constant $CaCl_2$ concentration: a) 0.5% (w/w); b) 2.75% (w/w); c) 5% (w/w).

The positive charge can be attributed to the chitosan coating on the surface of the particles. The dominant localization of chitosan in the particle wall was observed by imaging the chitosan-Ca-alginate particles with FITC-labeled chitosan using confocal laser scanning microscopy (Mladenovska et al., 2007a; 2007b).

Content of the cross-linking agent in the synbiotic microparticles

Calcium content in the synbiotic microparticles was used as a measure for mechanical and chemical stability of the obtained particles. Ca-content in the chitosan-Ca-alginate microparticles of different series ranged from 0.43-1.22 mg $Ca^{2+}$/10 mg particles (Table 1). In the experimental system, this response was analyzed similarly as the particle size, in conjunction with $CaCl_2$ and chitosan concentrations required to provide high probiotic viability in gastric juice and desirable zeta potential. The value of the regression coefficient $b_3$ points that the Ca-content is mostly affected by the $CaCl_2$ concentration, while the value of the coefficient $b_1$ indicates lower, but also significant effect of alginate concentration ($x_1$). The concentration of chitosan ($x_2$) does not affect the Ca-content of the microparticles significantly (Table 2). Increase in $CaCl_2$ concentration in the cross-linking medium increased Ca-content, while with increase in the alginate concentration, the Ca-content decreased. The best response for Ca-content was obtained at chitosan concentration 0.5% w/w in the experimental range of alginate 1-2% w/w and $CaCl_2$ 4.4-5% w/w. However, the findings that alginate concentration above 2.5% w/w is needed to provide sufficient probiotic viability in gastric pH and increase in alginate concentration from 1 to 4% w/w provides higher survival rate during microencapsulation were the main reasons for accepting the lower value as an optimum (0.94 mg $Ca^{2+}$/10 mg particles was obtained vs. predicted one 1.04 mg $Ca^{2+}$ /10 mg particles).

Viability of *L. casei* 01 after preparation of synbiotic microparticles

Simultaneous microencapsulation of prebiotics and probiotics results in synbiosis that may provide enhanced protection during preparation, storage and exposure to gastrointestinal conditions. In our previous study (Petreska Ivanovska et al., 2012a), higher survival for 4 logs was observed when *L. casei* 01 was spray-dried in the presence of alginate and FOS in comparison with the survival of the spray-dried *L. casei* 01 alone. There are other research data that point to increased viability of *L. casei* in a presence of FOSs with different degrees of polymerization (Aryana & McGrew, 2007; Ping et al., 2007). Moreover, FOS is effectively utilized by strains of *L. casei* to produce organic acids, such as lactic and acetic acid (Liong & Shah, 2005a, b), which may beneficially affect the human glucose and lipid metabolism. Having these in regard, the medium intended for spray-drying as well as the juice containing free cells was supplied with the prebiotic FOS, in addition to the probiotic.

In this research, the yield of the spray-drying process was 46.5±9.7, with viability of the probiotic after spray-drying from 7.78 log cfu/g to 11.76 log cfu/g within the different series of the experimental plan. In comparison with the spray-drying process, the loss of viability during freeze-drying was insignificant for all experimental series and viability of the probiotic in the microparticles after freeze-drying was between 7.26 log cfu/g and 11.30 log cfu/g (Table 1). This response was used as a key one for optimization of the formulation variables during the preparation of the microparticles. The viability of the microencapsulated *L. casei* 01 increases with increasing the concentrations of alginate and $CaCl_2$, while the concentration of chitosan negatively affects the probiotic viability. It was suggested chitosan to be used for additional coating of alginate beads due to the inhibitory effect of chitosan on different lactic acid bacteria (Zhou et al., 1998). However, according to the values of regression coefficients, $b_1$, $b_2$ and $b_3$ (Table 2), the viability of *L. casei* 01 in microparticles obtained after freeze-drying was mostly affected by the alginate ($x_1$) and $CaCl_2$ concentration ($x_3$), while the chitosan concentration had the lowest influence on this response. In order to investigate this response for the given experimental range and to define the optimal values of the formulation factors, contour diagrams for viability of L. casei 01 after freeze-drying was constructed (Fig. 4). The diagrams present the viability values as a function of alginate $(x_1)$ and $CaCl_2$ concentration $(x_3)$, while chitosan concentration $(x_2)$ was kept constant at 0.1% (w/w) (Fig. 4a), 0.3% (w/w) (Fig. 4b) and 0.5% (w/w) (Fig. 4c).

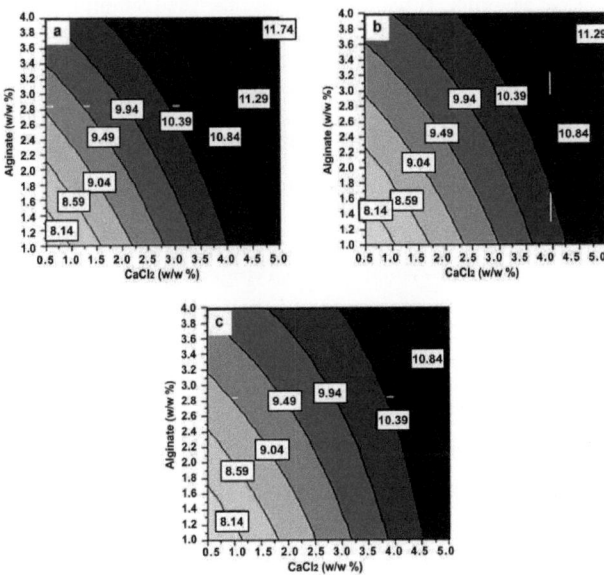

Figure 4. A contour diagrams of the viability of microencapsulated L. casei 01 after freeze-drying as a function of alginate and $CaCl_2$ concentrations at constant chitosan concentration: a) 0.1 (w/w %); b) 0.3 (w/w %); c) 0.5 (w/w %).

The best response for the probiotic viability was obtained at chitosan concentration of 0.1% w/w in the concentration range of alginate 1.87-4% w/w and $CaCl_2$ 3.85-5% w/w, however with no significant effect on the probiotic viability when increased chitosan concentration up to 0.5% w/w was used. Namely, equal or similar response for the probiotic viability was obtained at chitosan concentration of 0.3% (w/w) and 0.5% (w/w) for the experimental ranges of alginate 3.2–4% (w/w) and $CaCl_2$ 4.64–5% (w/w) (Fig. 4b), and 2.17–4% (w/w) and 4.29-5% (w/w) (Fig. 4c), respectively.

Chen et al., (2005) suggested that concentration of 1% for sodium alginate is an optimal for encapsulation of probiotics using an extrusion method and provides sufficient probiotic viability. It was also found that 1% sodium alginate did not provide enough protection for probiotics during storage and in simulated gastric fluid. Later, when investigating an optimal model for the encapsulating materials of probiotic microcapsules that provide sufficient viability after one week storage, it was confirmed that 3% sodium alginate with 1% peptides and 3% FOS was more appropriate for increasing probiotic viability after manufacturing, storage and gastric fluid test (Chen et al., 2006). In our study, in which spray-drying method was used, sodium alginate concentration higher than 1.87% should be utilized in order similar effects immediately after preparation to be achieved.

Viability of *L. casei* 01 in simulated gastrointestinal conditions

To estimate the influence of the formulation factors on the stability of the probiotic in gastrointestinal conditions, the viability of the microencapsulated *L. casei* 01 during incubation in simulated gastric and bile salt solutions was determined. Formulations generated with the experimental design demonstrated significantly different values for the viability of the encapsulated *L. casei* 01 in a range of 4.32-9.62 log cfu/g during incubation of the microparticles in simulated gastric juice with pH 1.5 (Table 1). The values of the coefficient $b_1$ and especially of $b_3$ (Table 2) demonstrate that the viability of the microencapsulated *L. casei* 01 in simulated gastric juice is dominantly affected by the alginate $(x_1)$ and $CaCl_2$ concentration $(x_3)$, with the latest factor as the most significant. The influence of the chitosan concentration was not significant and, in addition, no major interactions were found. We also observed that further increase in CaCl$_2$ concentration improves the probiotic viability in acidic pH, probably as a consequence of the increased degree of ionic cross-linking.

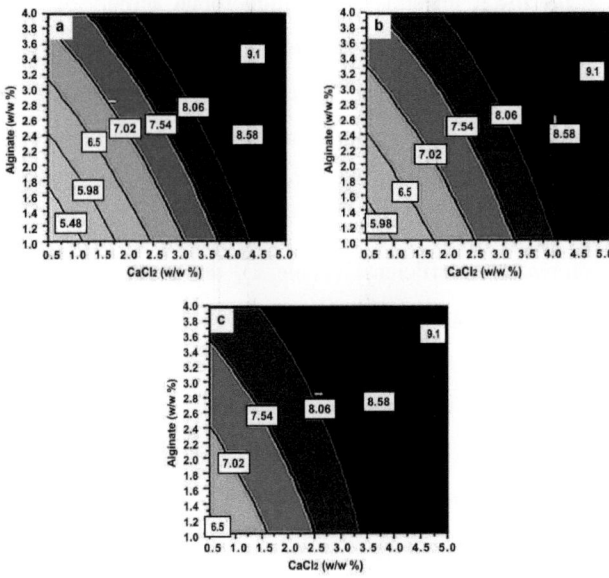

Figure 5. A contour diagrams of the viability of microencapsulated *L. casei* 01 in simulated gastric juice with pH 1.5 as a function of alginate and CaCl$_2$ concentrations at constant chitosan concentration: a) 0.1% w/w; b) 0.3% w/w; c) 0.5% w/w.


The contour diagrams at Fig. 5 present the viability of the microencapsulated *L. casei* 01 in simulated gastric juice as a function of alginate ($x_1$) and CaCl$_2$ concentration ($x_3$), while the concentration of chitosan ($x_2$) was kept constant at 0.1% w/w (Fig. 5a), 0.3% w/w (Fig. 5b) and 0.5% w/w (Fig. 5c). One can notice that the probiotic viability of at least 9.1 log cfu/g is predicted when alginate in concentration range of 2.64-4% w/w and CaCl$_2$ in concentration range of 4.64-5% w/w were used, with the concentration of chitosan maintained at 0.5% w/w (Fig. 5c), thus it was considered as an optimal response.

Further, it is well known that the viability of the probiotics is adversely affected by the bile salts in the lower intestine. The antimicrobial activity of the bile due to the dissolution of bacterial membranes disrupts the integrity of the cells. The protective effect of the prepared synbiotic microparticles in respect to the viability of *L. casei* 01 in intestinal juice was evaluated during additional 3 h in simulated intestinal juice (pH 6.8) with 1% bile salts. Significantly different values for the viability of encapsulated *L. casei* 01 in a range of 2.27-8.46 log cfu/g were observed (Table 1). Considering the values of the regression coefficients (Table 2), the probiotic viability in simulated intestinal juice was significantly affected by the concentration of $CaCl_2$ ($x_3$), while the two other factors, $x_1$ and $x_2$, showed almost equal effects. However, the lowest value of the coefficient $b_2$ indicates the lowest influence of the chitosan concentration on the investigated response. The values of interaction terms, $b_{12}$, $b_{13}$ and $b_{23}$ pointed to non-significant interactions between the formulation factors. At the optimum point of concentrations of the formulation factors (4% w/w alginate, 0.5% w/w chitosan and 5% w/w $CaCl_2$) high survival rate of *L. casei* 01 in intestinal juice, above 8 log cfu/g, was obtained (Table 1).

Effective colonization of the colon with viable and metabolically active probiotic cells is a crucial prerequisite for providing postulated health effects. Viability and/or release of microencapsulated *L. casei* 01 in simulated colon conditions were monitored in different time intervals up to 24 h of the initial incubation. Viability of microencapsulated *L. casei* 01 in simulated colon conditions (pH 7.4) ranged from non-viable cells to 8.31 log cfu/g (Table 1). All the investigated factors increased the probiotic viability in simulated colon conditions, while the best response for probiotic viability of 7.97 log cfu/g was obtained at alginate concentration (factor with the lowest effect) of 4% w/w in the concentration range of chitosan, 0.1-0.46% w/w and $CaCl_2$, 4.2-5% w/w.

Considering above-mentioned, the optimal formulation of synbiotic chitosan-Ca-alginate microparticles provides effective protection of the probiotic during exposure in simulated gastric juice ($9.62\pm0.1$ log cfu/g) and relatively high survival rate in intestinal juice with pH 6.8 ($8.46\pm0.2$ log cfu/g). In addition, the released cell count in colonic pH after 24 h exposure to simulated GI conditions was $7.67\pm0.4$ log cfu/g. We also observed that by increasing the concentration of the microencapsulating material, the survival rate of *L. casei* 01 increased and, under storage conditions, the viability maintained above the therapeutic level (6-7 log cfu/g). At the end of the 3 month-storage of the optimal formulation at 4 °C, viability of the probiotic cells was $8.1\pm0.6$ log cfu/g. Considering the viability data immediately after preparation ($11.3\pm0.5$ log cfu/g) and under refrigerated storage, the optimized microencapsulated synbiotic satisfied the recommendation for the effective dosage of $10^7–10^9$ cfu/100 mg probiotic products per day (Minelli & Benini, 2008). In addition, the physicochemical parameters of the optimal formulation, $d_{50}$ of $8.77\pm0.4$ μm, zeta potential of $21.56\pm1.1$ mV and Ca-content of $0.94\pm0.15$ mg/10 mg, point to the great potential for effective colonization of the probiotic in the lower intestine.

## 4.2 Physicochemical properties of the optimal formulation of synbiotic microparticles

Physicochemical characterization of the optimal formulation of synbiotic microparticles included morphological analysis before and after mechanical treatment of the particles (Fig. 6a, b), stability assay of the probiotic during microencapsulation (Fig. 7) and swelling properties of the prepared microparticles (Fig. 8).

Morphology of the synbiotic microparticles

The morphological analysis of the freeze-dried microparticles as we already reported (Petreska Ivanovska et al., 2012a) showed spherical shape with wrinkled surface resulted from the encapsulated cells and loss of water during spray- and freeze-drying processes.

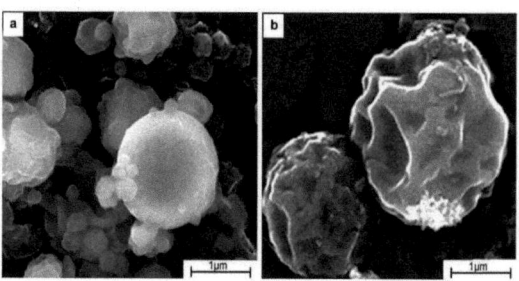

Figure 6. SEM of microparticles using high vacuum technique. (a) Intact chitosan-Ca-alginate microparticles; (b) *L. casei* 01 loaded chitosan-Ca-alginate microparticles scanned after mechanical treatment.

In this study, when intact microparticles were scanned, the wrinkles were not observed (Fig. 6a). In addition, tendency of the particles to agglomerate can be noticed, probably as a result of attractive electrostatic forces between the polymers.

The image obtained after mechanical treatment of the microparticles using high vacuum SEM clearly shows formation of certain invaginations on the surface of the microparticles with non-significant disruptions of the structure (Fig. 6b), thus, indicating that the microparticles may be further processed and/or applied in different food or pharmaceutical products.

Stability of *L. casei* 01 during microencapsulation

FTIR spectra are specific to a given bacterial strain and show spectral characteristics of cell components such as fatty acids, membrane and intracellular proteins, polysaccharides and nucleic acids (Vodnar et al., 2010). Thus, the FTIR spectroscopy may be used for rapid identification of the spectra pattern changes of probiotic cells during microencapsulation. In a view of the complex structure of the synbiotic chitosan-Ca-alginate microparticles, a rough assignment of the corrected FTIR-ATR spectra of *L. casei* 01, non-encapsulated and released from the microparticles, has been made (Fig. 7). Namely, two distinctive bands at ~2845 cm$^{-1}$ and ~2929 cm$^{-1}$ due to the asymmetric stretching of methyl and methylene groups, respectively, were detected. These bands are specific to the fatty acids of the wall of probiotic bacteria (Schmitt & Flemming, 1998). CH$_3$- and CH$_2$- asymmetric and symmetric deformations of proteins (~1430 cm$^{-1}$ and ~1372 cm$^{-1}$, respectively) (Filip & Hermann, 2001) were also detected. A band at ~1730 cm$^{-1}$ due to the C=O stretching vibration of the ester groups into the fatty acids and lipids together with Amide I and Amide II bands at ~1620 cm$^{-1}$ and 1530 cm$^{-1}$ from proteins were observed.

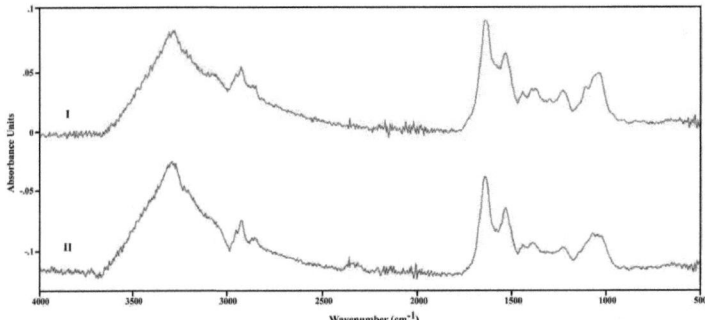

Figure 7. FTIR spectra of non-encapsulated *L. casei* 01 (I) and released from the synbiotic chitosan-Ca-alginate microparticles (II).

In the IR fingerprint region, the symmetric and asymmetric stretching from the phosphodiester component of the nucleic acids at 1030 $cm^{-1}$ and 1190 $cm^{-1}$ were found as well as the C-O-C deformation vibration from the polysaccharides (900-1200 $cm^{-1}$) bonded to the glycopeptides and lipopolysaccharides of the cell wall (Filip & Hermann, 2001). Almost identical features of the FTIR spectra of *L. casei* 01 released from the microparticles and non-encapsulated one suggested preserved stability of the probiotic cells during the microencapsulation process. In addition, both spectra included band at 1127 $cm^{-1}$ emerged from the lactic acid as a fermentation product.

Swelling studies

To confirm the targeted and controlled delivery function of the probiotic loaded chitosan-Ca-alginate microparticles, the swelling behavior of the optimal formulation was investigated in mediums with different pH values respective to simulated gastrointestinal conditions. An exchange method was used, where particles were firstly placed in medium with pH 1.5 for 3 h, then in pH 6.8 for additional 3 h and subsequently in pH 7.4 for 4 h. The results point that synbiotic microparticles have no significant tendency for swelling, especially in mediums with pH 1.5 and 6.8 where increase in $d_{50}$ of 12.26% and 31.62% (Fig. 8), respectively, was observed. The protection of probiotic cells encapsulated in chitosan-Ca-alginate microparticles was achieved by chemical cross-linking with $Ca^{2+}$ ions able to diffuse into the alginate gel network. Increased swelling degree of the microparticles in pH 7.4 was observed, with increase in $d_{50}$ for 54.89% (Fig. 8), probably due to the exchange of $Na^{+}$ with $Ca^{2+}$ ions when pH moves towards more alkaline pH and increased porosity and diffusion of the medium into the vicinity of the particles. Having in regard the morphologic characteristics of the chitosan-Ca-alginate microparticles i.e. low porosity and non-significant increase in particle size, especially in pH 1.5 and 6.8, one can conclude that the probiotic will be released in the lower intestine with the degradation of the microparticles as a dominant release mechanism.

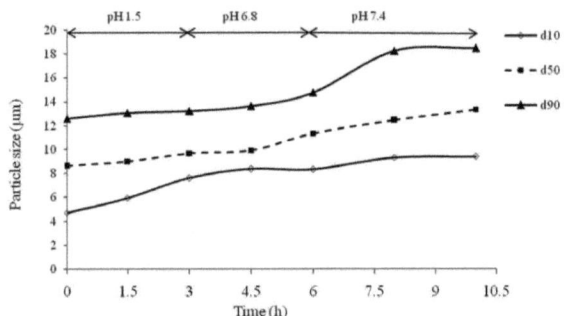

Figure 8. Effect of different pH values on the swelling behavior of synbiotic microparticles of the optimal formulation evaluated by size measurements of microparticles after incubation at pH 1.5, 6.8 and 7.4.

4.3 Incorporation of free and encapsulated synbiotic in carrot juice

Survival of free and encapsulated *L. casei* 01 in carrot juice during fermentation and storage

Certain beverages are quite acidic and best suited to fermentation by probiotic lactobacilli, but use of microencapsulation technology could aid in the delivery of viable probiotic cells (Champagne & Fustier, 2007). Thus, an optimal formulation of the synbiotic microparticles was used to prepare new functional beverages (fermented and non-fermented) that were compared with the properties of the functional juices containing non-encapsulated *L. casei* 01 and prebiotic FOS. The viability of free and encapsulated *L. casei* 01 in fermented samples after 24-h fermentation was 10.46±0.4 log cfu/ml and 9.6±0.3 log cfu/ml, respectively, from the starting cell count of 7.4±0.1

log cfu/ml (Fig. 9a). The bacterial growth is characterized by initial, exponential and stationary phase. In the initial phase, bacterial culture adapts to the medium followed by synthesis of enzymes need to utilize the available nutrients enabling multiplication and propagation of the cells. The most proliferative phase is the exponential one, when maximal biomass is accumulated in the medium. Simultaneously, the amount of the nutrients declines, while the production of growth inhibitory metabolites tends to increase and the cells enter in the stationary phase of their growth. During the fermentation process, free probiotic cells of *L. casei* 01 efficiently utilized carrot juice as an energy source. In addition, lactic acid fermentation of carrot juice has been found to positively influence the availability of certain minerals like Ca, P and Fe, β-carotene, betaine and vitamin C (Rakin et al., 2007). Rapid and continuous growth of *L. casei* NRRL B-442 during 24-h fermentation in cashew apple juice has been documented by Pereira et al., (2011). *L. casei* ATCC 393 also grew well during fermentation at 37 °C for 72 h in potato juice without nutrient supplementation (Kim et al., 2012). Kun et al., (2008) reported enormous increase in viable bifidobacteria strains (*B. lactis* Bb-12, B. *bifidum* B7.1 and B3.2) in inoculated carrot juice, but only for the first 12 h of the fermentation when survival rate started to decline upon 24-th hour of fermentation. Carrot juice was not a promising carrier for *B. lactis* 420 and *B. lactis* Bb-12 since these bacteria did not grow during overnight fermentation at 37 °C (Tamminen et al., 2013). In the same study, almost unchanged viability of $10^9 - 10^{10}$ cfu/ml during 4 weeks storage of fermented carrot juice, which declined only to $10^6 - 10^7$ cfu/ml after 12 weeks storage, was found for the strains *L. plantarum* Lp-115, *L. rhamnosus* GG and *L. paracasei* Lpc-37. Considerable number of *Lactobacillus* sp. have been shown to successfully ferment various vegetable juices including cabbage, beet, pumpkin, courgette and carrot juices supplemented with prebiotics (Martins et al., 2013).

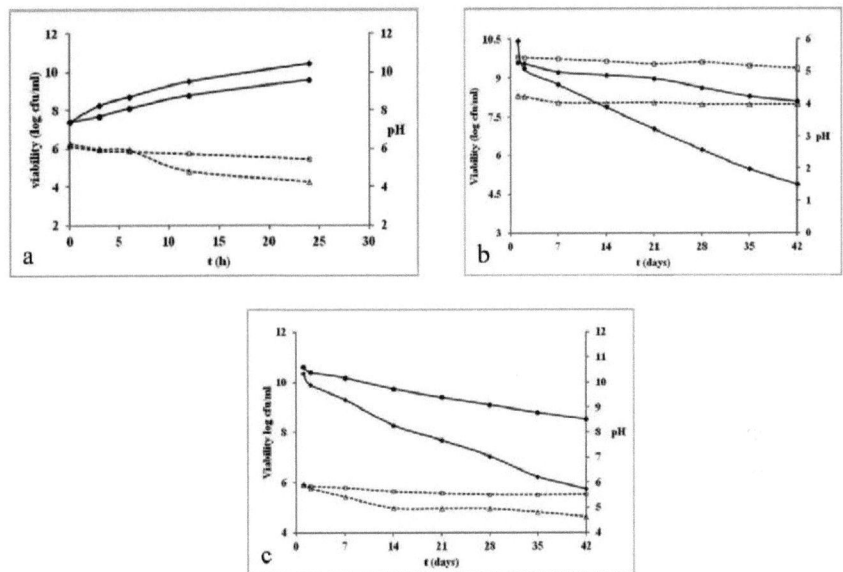

Figure 9. Changes in viability (whole line) of free (♦) and microencapsulated *L. casei* 01 (●) and pH values (interrupted line) of free cells juice (Δ) and juice with encapsulated *L. casei* 01 (□) during fermentation of carrot juice (a), cold storage of fermented carrot juice (b) and non-fermented juice (c).

Encapsulated *L. casei* 01 in our fermentation test grew well, however showed slightly lower cell count compared to the juice containing free cells. The selective permeability of the chitosan-alginate membrane (Anal & Stevens, 2005) may explain the delayed growth of the encapsulated cells. Opposite to our finding, Nazzaro et al., (2009) investigated the fermentative ability of alginate-xanthan-inulin encapsulated *L. acidophilus* and revealed significantly higher viability of the encapsulated probiotic after 48-h fermentation of the carrot juice. Similar results have been reported by King et al.,

45

(2007) during 80-h fermentation of tomato juice with immobilized cells of *L. acidophilus*.

At the end of the fermentation period, the pH value of the juice inoculated with free cells was found to be lower than that of the microparticles added juice, 4.26 and 5.45, respectively (Fig. 9a). The reduction of pH in the carrot juice from the initial value of 6.25±0.1 is expected due to the saccharolytic activity of lactic acid bacteria.

Probiotics are known to utilize sugars degraded upon action of the secreted carbohydrase followed by production of lactic acid. Research data pointed to the conclusion that FOS with low molecular weight is better utilized by *L. casei* 01 followed by pH reduction of the medium to approximately 4, while there are strains which cannot ferment FOS and decrease pH slightly below 6 (Kaplan & Hutkins, 2000). Having these findings in regard, one can conclude that FOS as a prebiotic is successfully fermented by *L. casei* 01 and its utilization as a source of energy for the growth of free cells is significantly higher comparing to encapsulated cells. In contrast to the observations during the fermentation process, the viable cell counts of microencapsulated *L. casei* 01 in fermented carrot juice was 8.1±0.13 log cfu/ml after 6 weeks of cold storage at 4 °C, while that of free cells was only 4.89±0.1 log cfu/ml (Fig. 9b), which confirms the role of the microencapsulation in improving probiotic viability. Moreover, the pH values of the synbiotic carrot juice with free cells were lower than pH values of carrot juice with microencapsulated cells during all investigation period, which might negatively affect the sensory properties of the product (Fig. 9b).

Survival of free and encapsulated *L. casei* 01 in non-fermented carrot juice

During 6 weeks storage at 4 °C, the viability of *L. casei* 01 in non-fermented synbiotic carrot juices with free and microencapsulated cells was also investigated. Microencapsulated cells survive better than free cells in carrot juice, with viable cell counts of 8.52±0.2 log cfu/ml and 5.74±0.11 log cfu/ml after storage, respectively (Fig.

9c). Ding & Shah (2008) have also found that encapsulated probiotic cells survived in orange and apple juices throughout the 6 weeks of storage, while free cells lost their viability within 5 weeks and confirmed that the fruit juices containing microencapsulated probiotic bacteria are more stable than those containing free cells. On the contrary, Champagne & Gardner (2008) have been reported viability of *L. rhamnosus*, *L. plantarum*, *L. reuteri* and *L. fermentum* incorporated in several commercial fruit drinks to be above 6 log cfu/ml during 80-days of storage at 4 °C. In our study, free cells were in therapeutically accepted range upon fifth week of storage, whereas encapsulated showed better resistance to the end of the assay. In addition, significant reduction in pH (1.56 units) in free cells juice was noticed, while in synbiotic carrot juice containing encapsulated cells, lower decline of pH (0.62 units) was observed. This result confirmed that the chitosan-Ca-alginate matrix could protect probiotic cells by buffering the acidic environment to which probiotic is exposed. Whey protein isolate (WPI) matrix or WPI in combination with a physically-modified resistant starch was also effective to preserve the viability of spray-dried microencapsulated *L. rhamnosus* GG in apple juice or citrate buffer (pH 3.5) (Ying et al., 2012). Further, the protective effect of these matrices was found to be higher compared to the formulation containing resistant starch alone due to the ability of WPI to create a buffered local microenvironment within the hydrated colloid particle surrounding the encapsulated *L. rhamnosus* GG and isolating the bacteria from the stress of the acidic environment.

Short chain organic acid profile of synbiotic carrot juice during fermentation and storage

Probiotic bacteria may utilize carbohydrates and produce small amounts of organic acids, thus, their metabolic activity can be estimated by the production of lactic and acetic acid. Capability of probiotic bacteria to ferment carbohydrates available in the growth medium in general and in this respect in fruit and vegetable juices depends on

47

the bacterial strain itself, but also on the type of the nutrients, growth promoters and inhibitors, osmotic pressure, inoculum size, fermentation period and storage temperature (Shah, 2000). The concentrations of lactic and acetic acid in carrot juice alone were 0.05 mg/ml and 0.13 mg/ml, respectively. Fig. 10a illustrates the lactic and acetic acid concentration in carrot juice containing free and microencapsulated *L. casei* 01 during fermentation. The production of lactic and acetic acid tends to increase during 24-h fermentation with enhanced production in juice containing encapsulated cells upon 12 h. Further, it is clearly presented that the production of acetic acid in juice containing encapsulated cells was slightly increased to the end of the fermentation, while the concentration of lactic acid was dramatically increased in free cells juice after 12-h fermentation. At the end of fermentation, the respective values for the concentrations of lactic and acetic acid were $2.75\pm0.03$ and $0.27\pm0.01$ mg/ml in free cells juice and $1.66\pm0.04$ and $0.52\pm0.01$ mg/ml for the juice with encapsulated cells, respectively. Increased production of lactic and acetic acid during fermentation due to the bacterial growth is accompanied with organic acid accumulation. Lactic acid increases nutritional value of fermented products by engendering their taste. In addition, it has significant role in maintaining proton moving force of bacterial cells and in absence of carbohydrates, some of bacteria utilize it as an energy source. Moreover, the high content of mineral components in carrot juice may improve the lactic acid fermentation. As the metabolism pathway of lactic acid bacteria lead to the production of lactic acid mainly, the high ratio in the favour of produced lactic acid during the fermentation of carrot juice with *L. casei* 01 is reasonable. Increased growth of free *L. casei* 01 during our fermentation assay (Fig. 9a) explains the higher lactic acid production compared to the juice containing encapsulated cells.

The significantly lower amount of acetic acid produced is also expected. However, the production of acetic acid in the juice containing microparticles is probably stimulated by carboxylic groups of the alginate that become protonated in the acidic medium

(Doumeche et al., 2004). Although, acetic acid is responsible for the sour taste of the juice, its antimicrobial properties improve the functional value of the product.

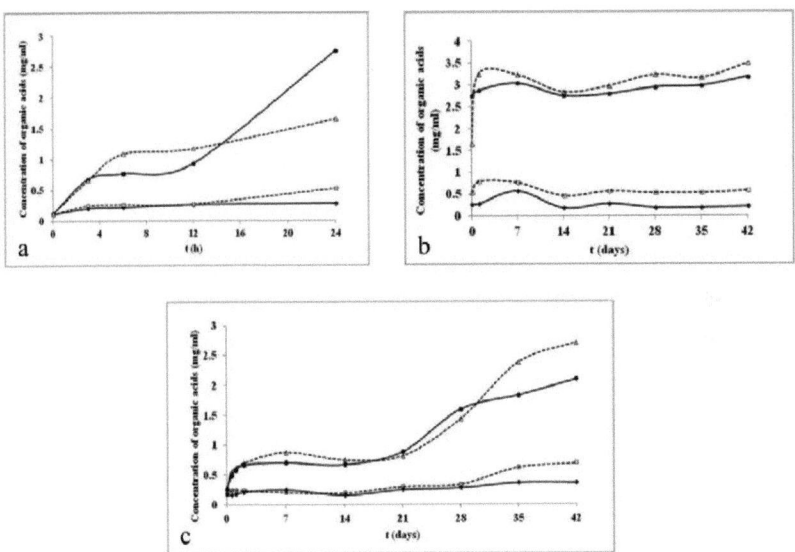

Figure 10. Production of lactic acid (•, Δ) and acetic acid (♦, □) during fermentation of carrot juice (a), storage of fermented carrot juice (b) and non-fermented juice (c) with free cells (whole line) and microencapsulated *L. casei* 01 (interrupted line).

The amount of acetic acid during 6 weeks of refrigerated storage of fermented samples containing free cells as well encapsulated ones was at constant level albeit certain fluctuations of the concentration were determined. Thus, the acetic acid content decreased from 0.27 to 0.21 mg/ml in free cells juice, while in the juice containing encapsulated cells, it slightly increased from 0.52 to 0.57 mg/ml. In contrast, the amount of lactic acid tends to increase during the storage period, especially in the juice containing encapsulated cells with enhancement of the production of 1.66 to 3.49 mg/ml (Fig. 10b). Increase in the amount of lactic acid in carrot juice containing microparticles in storage conditions is probably due to the gradual leakage of the encapsulated cells from the chitosan-Ca-alginate matrix in the medium and slower utilization of the substrate. Although, the level of organic acids in the fermented juice containing free cells remained stable after 6 weeks of cold storage, the progressive cell loss pointed to the microencapsulation as the effective tool to preserve metabolically active cells.

Short chain organic acid profile of non-fermented synbiotic carrot juice during storage

According to the survival rate of *L. casei* 01 in non-fermented synbiotic carrot juices during 6 weeks of cold storage, the analysis of organic acids showed that higher amount was produced in juice containing synbiotic microparticles, 2.7 and 0.69 mg/ml for lactic and acetic acid, respectively, while in free cells juice the respective quantities were 2.1 and 0.37 mg/ml (Fig. 10c). The results indicated that *L. casei* 01 cells retained its metabolic activity, even in the cold storage conditions without prior fermentation at 37 °C. Increased amount of lactic and acetic acids in juice containing encapsulated *L. casei* 01 confirmed the effective preservation of the active probiotic cells by the microencapsulation method used in this study.

10. CONCLUSION

In this study, synbiotic loaded chitosan-Ca-alginate microparticles were prepared and subsequently incorporated in functional carrot juice. The processing conditions and optimal formulation of the synbiotic loaded microparticles, prepared of 4% w/w alginate, 0.5% w/w chitosan and 5% w/w $CaCl_2$, provide stability of the probiotic *L. casei* 01 after microencapsulation and viability high above therapeutic minimum during preparation, storage and incubation of synbiotic microparticles in simulated gastric and intestinal juice, with efficient release of viable and metabolically active probiotic cells able to grow and colonize the lower intestine. The viability of the microencapsulated probiotic cells was also preserved when they were incorporated in functional carrot juice and their metabolic activity was also confirmed through production of organic acids. Considering that and the physicochemical properties of the optimal formulation of synbiotic microparticles, one can say that the carrot juice containing synbiotic microparticles may be a new functional product with satisfactory sensorial profile. However, the consumers' acceptance of this functional carrot juice should be further studied. Although low in size, the synbiotic microparticles tend to agglomerate and sediment, which may affect the textural quality of the carrot juice. In addition, the synergistic effect of the prebiotic FOS on the probiotic viability and the potential of this functional beverage to deliver the probiotic effectively in the lower intestine as well as to exert beneficiary health effects have to be confirmed in *in vivo* studies.

## 11. ACKNOWLEDGMENTS

This research was financially supported by the Ministry of Education and Science of the Republic of Macedonia (Project No. 08-99). The authors would like to thank IMCD (UK) for the donation of sodium alginate (Protanal 10/60 LS, FMC BioPolymer, USA). Gratitude is expressed also to the University of Reading, Centre for Advanced Microscopy, United Kingdom, for providing SEM images of the synbiotic microparticles.

# 12. REFERENCE

Almansa C., Agrawal A., Houghton L.A., Intestinal microbiota, patophysiology and translation to probiotic use in patients with irritable bowel syndrome. Expert Rev. Gastroenterol. Hepatol. 6(3): 383-398 (2012).

Anal A.K., Stevens W.F., Chitosan-alginate multilayer beads for controlled release of ampicillin. Int. J. Pharm. 290: 45-54 (2005).

Anal A., Singh H., Recent advances in microencapsulation of probiotics for industrial applications and targeted delivery. Trends Food Sci. Technol. 18: 240-251 (2007).

Anekella K., Orsat V., Optimization of microencapsulation of probiotics in raspberry juice by spray drying. LWT-Food Sci. Technol. 50: 17-24 (2013).

Aryana K.J., McGrew P., Quality attributes of yogurt with *L. casei* and various prebiotics. LWT-Food Sci. Technol. 40: 1808-1814 (2007).

Birkett A.M., Francis C.C., Short-chain fructo-oligosaccharide: a low molecular weight fraction. In Cho S.S., Finocchiaro E.T., (Edit.). Handbook of Prebiotics and Probiotics Ingredients. CRC Press Taylor & Francis Group, Boca Raton, Florida, p: 13-42 (2010).

Burgain J., Gaiani C., Linder M., Scher J., Encapsulation of probiotic living cells: from laboratory scale to industrial applications. J. Food Eng. 104: 467-483 (2011).

Casiraghi M.C., Canzi E., Zanchi R., Donati E., Villa L., Effects of a synbiotic milk product on human intestinal ecosystem. J. Appl. Microbiol. 103(2): 499-506 (2007).

Castro F.P., Cunha T.M., Ogliari P.J., Teófilo R.F., Ferreira M.M.C., Prudêncio E.S., Influence of different content of cheese whey and oligofructose on the properties of fermented lactic beverages: Study using response surface methodology. LWT-Food Sci. Technol. 42: 993-997 (2009a).

Castro F.P., Cunha T.M., Barreto P.L.M., Amboni R.D.M.C., Prudêncio E.S., Effect of oligofructose incorporation on the properties of fermented probiotic lactic beverages. Int. J. Dairy Technol. 62: 74-82 (2009b).

Ceapa C., Wopereis H., Rezaïki L., Kleerebezem M., Knol J., Oozeer R., Influence of fermented milk products, prebiotics and probiotics on microbiota composition and health. Best Pract. Res. Clin. Gastroenterol. 27(1): 139-155 (2013).

Chaikham P., Apichartsrangkoon A., Jirarattanarangsri W., Van de Wiele T., Influence of encapsulated probiotics combined with pressurized longan juice on colon microflora and their metabolic activities on the exposure to simulated dynamic gastrointestinal tract. Food Res. Int. 49: 133-142 (2012).

Champagne C.P., Gardner N.J., Roy D., Challenges in the addition of probiotic cultures to foods. Crit. Rev. Food Sci. Nutr. 45: 61-84 (2005).

Champagne C.P., Fustier P., Microencapsulation for the improved delivery of bioactive compounds into foods. Curr. Opin. Biotechnol. 18: 184-190 (2007).

53

Champagne C.P., Gardner N.J., Effect of storage in a fruit drink on subsequent survival of probiotic lactobacilli to gastro-intestinal stresses. Food Res. Int. 41: 539-543 (2008).

Chávarri M., Marañón A., Ares R., Ibáñez F.C., Marzo F., del Carmen Villarán M., Microencapsulation of a probiotic and prebiotic in alginate-chitosan capsules improves survival in simulated gastro-intestinal conditions. Int. J. Food Microbiol. 142: 185-189 (2010).

Chen K.N., Chen M.J., Liu J.R., Lin C.W., Chiu H.Y., Optimization of incorporated prebiotics as coating materials for probiotic microencapsulation. J. Food Sci. 70: 260-266 (2005).

Chen K.N., Chen M.J., Lin C.W., Optimal combination of the encapsulating materials for probiotic microcapsules and its experimental verification (R1). J. Food Eng. 76: 313-320 (2006).

Chen S., Cao Y., Ferguson L.R., Shu Q., Garg S., Evaluation of mucoadhesive coatings of chitosan and thiolated chitosan for the colonic delivery of microencapsulated probiotic bacteria. J. Microencapsul. 30(2): 103-115 (2013).

Cook M.T., Tzortzis G., Charalampopoulos D., Khutoryanskiy V.V., Microencapsulation of probiotics for gastrointestinal delivery. J. Control. Release 162: 56-67 (2012).

Corcoran B.M., Ross R.P., Fitzgerald G.F., Stanton C., Comparative survival of probiotic lactobacilli spray-dried in the presence of prebiotic substances. J. Appl. Microbiol. 96: 1024-1039 (2004).

Cui J.-H., Goh J.-S., Park S.-Y., Kim P.-H., Lee B.-J., Preparation and physical characterization of alginate microparticles using air atomization method. Drug Dev. Ind. Pharm. 27: 309-319 (2001).

Debon J., Prudêncio E.S., Petrus J.C.C., Fritzen-Freire C.B., Müler C.M.O., Amboni R.D.M.C., Vieira C.R.W., Storage stability of prebiotic fermented milk obtained from permeates resulting of the microfiltration process. LWT-Food Sci. Technol. 47: 96-102 (2012).

de Vrese M., Schrezenmeir J., Probiotics, prebiotics, and synbiotics. Adv. Biochem. Engin./Biotechnol. 111: 1-66 (2008).

Ding W.K., Shah N.P., Survival of free and microencapsulated probiotic bacteria in orange and apple juices. Int. Food Res. J. 15(2): 219-232 (2008).

Do Espírito Santo A.P., Perego P., Converti A., Oliveira M.N., Influence of food matrices on probiotic viability – A review focusing on the fruity bases. Trends Food Sci. Technol. 22(7): 377-385 (2011).

Doherty S.B., Gee V.L., Ross R.P, Stanton C., Fitzgerald G.F., Brodkorb A., Efficacy of whey protein gel networks as potential viability-enhancing scaffolds for cell immobilization of *Lactobacillus rhamnosus* GG. J. Microbiol. Methods 80: 231-241 (2010).

Doumeche B., Kuppers M., Stapf S., Blumich B., Hartmeier H., Ansorge-Schumacher B., New approaches to the visualization, quantification and explanation of acid-induced water loss from Ca-alginate hydrogel beads. J. Microencapsul. 21: 565-573 (2004).

Duncan S.H., Barcenilla A., Stewart C.S., Pryde S.E., Flint H.J., Acetate utilization and butyryl coenzyme A (CoA), acetate CoA transferase in butyrate producing bacteria from the human large intestine. Appl. Environ. Microbiol. 68: 5186-5190 (2002).

El-Gibaly I., Development and in vitro evaluation of novel floating chitosan microcapsules for oral use: comparison with non-floating chitosan microspheres. Int. J. Pharm. 249: 7-21 (2002).

FAO/WHO. Guidelines for the Evaluation of Probiotics in Food. Food and Agriculture Organization of United Nations and World Health Organization Working Group report, London, Ontario (2001).

FAO/WHO. Guidelines for the evaluation of probiotics in food. Joint FAO/WHO Working Group Report on Drafting Guidelines for the Evaluation of Probiotics in Food, London, Ontario (2002).

Favaro Trindade C.S., Heinemann R.J.B., Pedroso D.L., Developments in probiotic encapsulation. CAB Rev. Perspect. Agricult. Vet. Sci. Nutr. Nat. Resour. 6: 1-8 (2011).

Filip Z., Hermann S., An attempt to differentiate *Pseudomonas sp.* and other soil bacteria by FT-IR spectroscopy. Eur. J. Soil Biol. 37: 137-143 (2001).

Fritzen-Freire C.B., Prudêncio E.S., Amboni R.D.M.C., Pinto S.S., Negrão-Murakami A.N., Murakami F.S., Microencapsulation of bifidobacteria by spray drying in the presence of prebiotics. Food Res. Int. 45: 306-312 (2012).

Fujimori S., Gudis K., Mitsui K., Seo T., Yonezawa M., Tanaka S., Tatsuguchi A., Sakamoto C., A randomized controlled trial on the efficacy of synbiotic versus probiotic or prebiotic treatment to improve the quality of life in patients with ulcerative colitis. Nutrition 25: 520-525 (2009).

Gbassi G.K., Vandamme T., Probiotic encapsulation technology: from microencapsulation to release into gut. Pharmaceutics 4: 149-163 (2012).

Gentschew L., Ferguson L.R., Role of nutrition and microbiota in susceptability in inflammatory bowel disease. Mol. Nutr. Food Res. 56(4): 524-535 (2012).

Gibson G.R., Roberfroid M.B., Dietary modulation of the human colonic microflora: introducing the concept of prebiotics. J. Clin. Nutr. 125: 1401–1412 (1995).
Gibson G.R., Fibre and effects on probiotics (the prebiotic concept). Clin. Nutr. Suppl. 1: 25-31 (2004).

Gill H., Prasad J., Probiotics, immunomodulation, and health benefits. Adv. Exp. Med. Biol. 606: 423-454 (2008).

Gobbetti M., Di Cagno R., De Angelis M., Functional microorganisms for functional food quality. Crit. Rev. Food Sci. Nutr. 50: 716-727 (2010).

Gotteland M., Andrews M., Toledo M., Munoz L., Caceres P., Anziani A., Wittig E., Speisky H., Salazar G., Modulation of *Helicobacter pylori* colonization with cranberry juice and *Lactobacillus johnsonii* La1 in children. Nutrition 24(5): 421-426 (2008).

Granato D., Branco G.F., Cruz A.G., Faria J.A.F., Shah N.P., Probiotic dairy products as functional foods. Compr. Rev. Food Sci. Food Safety 9: 455-470 (2010).

Guarner F., Impacts of prebiotics on the immune system and inflammation. In: Calder, P.C., Yagoob, P., (Edit.). Diet Immunity and Inflammation. Woodhead Publishing, 11: 292-312 (2013).

Guergoletto K.B., Magnani M., San Martin J., Tardeli de Jesus Andrade C.G., Garcia S., Survival of *Lactobacillus casei* (LC-1) adhered to prebiotic vegetal fibers. Innov. Food Sci. Emerg. Technol. 11: 415-421 (2009).

Huebner J., Wehling, R.L., Hutkins R.W., Functional activity of commercial prebiotics. Int. Dairy J. 17: 770-775 (2007).

Huynh H.Q., deBruyn J., Guan L., Diaz H., Li M., Girgis S., Turner J., Fedorak R., Madsen K., Probiotic preparation VSL#3 induces remission in children with mild to moderate acute ulcerative colitis: a pilot study. Inflamm. Bowel Dis. 15(5): 760-768 (2009).

Kaplan H., Hutkins R.W., Fermentation of fructooligosaccharides by lactic-acid bacteria and bifidobacteria. Appl. Environ. Microbiol. 66: 2682-2684 (2000).

Khutoryanskiy V.V., Advances in mucoadhesion and mucoadhesive polymers. Macromol. Biosci. 11(6): 748-764 (2011).

Kılıç G.B., Highlights in Probiotic Research. In: Kongo, M. (Edit.). Lactic Acid Bacteria - R & D for Food, Health and Livestock Purposes. InTech, DOI: 10.5772/50004 (2013).

Kim N.J., Jang H.L., Yoon K.Y., Potato juice fermented with Lactobacillus casei as a probiotic functional beverage. Food Sci. Biotechnol. 21(5): 1301-1307 (2012).

King V.A.-E., Huang H.-Y., Tsen J.-H., Fermentation of tomato juice by cell immobilized *Lactobacillus acidophilus*. Mid-Taiwan J. Med. 12: 1-7 (2007).

Krinsky N.I., Johnson E.J., Carotenoid actions and their relation to health and disease. Mol. Aspects Med. 26: 459-516 (2005).

Kukkonen K., Savilahti E., Haahtela T., Probiotics and prebiotic galacto-oligosaccharides in the prevention of allergic diseases: a randomized, double-blined, placebo controlled trial. J. Allergy Clin. Immunol. 119: 192-198 (2007).

Kun S., Rezessy-Szabo J.M., Nguyen Q.D., Hoschke A., Changes of microbial population and some components in carrot juice during fermentation with selected *Bifidobacterium* strains. Process Biochem. 43: 816-821 (2008).

Liong M.T., Shah N.P., Optimization of cholesterol removal by probiotics in the presence of prebiotics by using a response surfase method. Appl. Environ. Microbiol. 71: 1745-1753 (2005a).

Liong M.T., Shah N.P., Optimization of growth of *Lactobacillus casei ASCC* 292 and production of organic acids in the presence of fructooligosaccharides and maltodextrin. J. Food Sci. 70: M113-M120 (2005b).

Livney Y.D., Milk proteins as vehicles for bioactives. Curr. Opin. Colloid Interface Sci. 15: 73-83 (2010).

López-Rubio A., Sanchez E., Wilkanowicz S., Sanz Y., Lagaron J.M., Electrospinning as a useful technique for the encapsulation of living *bifidobacteria* in food hydrocolloids. Food Hydrocolloid. 28: 159-167 (2012).

Luckow T., Delahanty C., Which juice is 'healthier'? A consumer study of probiotic non-dairy juice drinks. Food Qual. Prefer. 15: 751-759 (2004a).

Luyer M.D., Buurman W.A., Hadfoune M., Speelmans G., Knol J., Jacobs J.A., Dejong C.H.C., Vriesema A.J.M., Greve J.W.M., Strain specific effects of probiotics on gut barrier integrity following hemorrhagic shock. Infect. Immun. 73(6): 3689-3692 (2005).

Macfarlane S., Macfarlane G.T., Cummings J.H., Prebiotics in the gastrointestinal tract. Aliment. Pharmacol. Ther. 24: 701-714 (2006).

Macfarlane G.T., Steed H., Macfarlane S., Bacterial metabolism and health-related effects of galacto-oligosaccharides and other prebiotics. J. Appl. Microbiol. 104: 305-344 (2008).

Mandal S., Puniya A.K., Sing K., Effect of alginate concentracions on survival of microencapsulated *Lactobacillus casei* NCDC-298. Int. Dairy J. 16: 1190-1195 (2006).

Manojlović V., Nedović V.A., Kailasapathy K., Zuidam N.J., Encapsulation of probiotics for use in food products. In: Zuidam, N.J., Nedović, V.A. (Edit.). Encapsulation Technologies for Active Food Ingredients and Food Processing. Springer, New York, p: 269-302 (2010).

Marteau P.R., de Vrese M., Cellier C.J., Schrezenmeir J., Protection from gastrointestinal diseases with the use of probiotics. Am. J. Clin. Nutr. 73: 430S-436S (2001).

Marteau P., Seksik P., Jian R., Probiotics and intestinal health effects: a clinical perspective. Br. J. Nutr. (Suppl. S1), 88: S51-S57 (2002).

Martins E.M.F., Ramos A.M., Vanzela E.S.L., Stringheta P.C., de Oliveira Pinto C.L., Martins J.M., Products of vegetable origin: a new alternative for the consumption of probiotic bacteria. Food Res. Int. 51(2): 764-770 (2013).

Menshutina N.V., Gordienko M.G., Voinovskiy A.A., Zbicinski I., Spray drying of probiotics: process development and scale-up. Dry Technol. 28: 1170-1177 (2010).

Minelli S.E.B., Benini A., Relationship between number of bacteria and their probiotic effects. Microb. Ecol. Health Dis. 20: 180-183 (2008).

Mitropoulou G., Nedovic V., Goyal A., Kourkoutas Y., Immobilization technologies in probiotic food production. J. Nutr. Metab. 1-15 (2013), ID 716861.

Mladenovska K., Raicki R.S., Janevik E.I., Ristoski T., Pavlova M.J., Kavrakovski Z., Dodov M.G., Goracinova K., Colon-specific delivery of 5-aminosalicylic acid from chitosan-Ca-alginate microparticles. Int. J. Pharm. 342: 124-136 (2007a).
Mladenovska K., Cruaud O., Richomme P., Belamie E., Raicki R.S., Venier-Julienne M.-C., Popovski E., Benoit J.P., Goracinova K., 5-ASA loaded chitosan-Ca-alginate microparticles: Preparation and physicochemical characterization. Int. J. Pharm. 345: 59-69 (2007b).

Mokarram R.R., Mortazavi S.A., Najafi M.B.H., Shahidi F., The influemce of multi stage alginate coating on survivability of potential probiotic bacteria in simultated gastric and intestinal juice. Food Res. Int. 42(8): 1040-1045 (2009).

Nazzaro F., Fratianni F., Coppola R, Sada A., Orlando P., Fermentative ability of alginate-prebiotic encapsulated *Lactobacillus acidophilus* and survival under simulated gastrointestinal conditions. J. Funct. Foods I: 319-323 (2009).

Nualkaekul S., Charalampopoulos D., Survival of *Lactobacillus plantarum* in model solutions and fruit juices. Int. J. Food Microbiol. 146(2): 111-117 (2011).

Nualkaekul S., Deepika G., Charalampopoulos D., Survival of freeze dried *Lactobacillus plantarum* in instant fruit powders and reconstituted fruit juices. Food Res. Int. 48: 627-633 (2012).

Oliveira R.P.S., Florence A.C.R., Silva R.C., Perego P., Converti A., Gioeilli A.L., Oliveira M.N., Effect of different prebiotics on the fermentation kinetics, probiotic survival and fatty acids profiles in non-fat synbiotic fermented milk. Int. J. Food Microbiol. 128(3): 467-472 (2009).

Oliveira R.P.S., Perego P., Oliveira M.N., Converti A., Effect of inulin as prebiotic and synbiotic interactions between probiotics to improve fermented milk firmness. J. Food Eng. 10: 36-40 (2011a).

Oliveira R.P.S., Perego P., Oliveira M.N., Converti A., Effect of inulin as a prebiotic to improve growth and counts of a probiotic cocktail in fermented skim milk. LWT-Food Sci. Technol. 44(2): 520-523 (2011b).

O'Riordan K., Andrews D., Buckle K., Conway P., Evaluation of microencapsulation of a *Bifidobacterium* strain with starch as an approach to prolonging viability during storage. J. Appl. Microbiol. 91: 1059-1066 (2001).

Orlando A., Russo F., Intestinal microbiota, probiotics and human gastrointestinal cancers. J. Gastrointest. Cancer 44(2): 121-131 (2012).

Ouwehand A.C., Lagström H., Suomalainen T., Salminen S., Effect of probiotics on constipation, fecal azoreductase activity and fecal mucin content in the elderly. Ann. Nutr. Metab. 46(3-4): 159-162 (2002).

Pedroso D.L., Thomazini M., Heinemann R.J.B., Favaro-Trindade C.S., Protection of *Bifidobacterium lactis* and *Lactobacillus acidophilus* by microencapsulation using spray-chilling. Int. Dairy J. 26: 127-132 (2012).

Pelletier C., Bouley C., Cayuela C., Bouttier S., Bourlioux P., Bellon-Fontaine M.-N., Cell surface characteristics of *Lactobacillus casei* subsp. *casei*, *Lactobacillus paracasei* subsp. *paracasei*, and *Lactobacillus rhamnosus* strains. Appl. Environ. Microbiol. 63: 1725-1731 (1997).

Pereira A.L.F., Maciel T.C., Rodrigues S., Probiotic beverage from cashew apple juice fermented with *Lactobacillus casei*. Food Res. Int. 44(5): 1276-1283 (2011).

Petreska Ivanovska T., Petrushevska-Tozi L., Dabevska Kostoska M., Geshkovski N., Grozdanov A., Stain C. Stafilov T., Mladenovska K., Microencapsulation of *L. casei* in chitosan-Ca-alginate microparticles using spray-drying method. Mac. J. Chem.Chem. Eng. 31(1): 115-123 (2012a).

Petreska Ivanovska T., Petrushevska-Tozi L., Grozdanov A., Petkovska R., Hadjieva J., Popovski E., Stafilov T., Mladenovska K., From optimization of synbiotic microparticles prepared by spray-drying to development of new functional carrot juice. Chem. Ind. Chem. Eng. Quart. 20(4): 549-564 (2014a).

Petreska Ivanovska T., Smilkov K., Zhivikj Z., Petrushevska-Tozi L., Mladenovska K., Comparative evaluation *of viability of* encapsulated *Lactobacillus casei* using two different methods of microencapsulation. Int. J. Pharm. Phytopharmacol. Res. 4(1): 20-24 (2014b).

Petrović T., Nedović V., Dimitrijević-Branković S., Bugarski B., Lacroix C., Protection of probiotic microorganisms by microencapsulation. Chem. Ind. Chem Eng. Quart. 13(3): 169-174 (2007).

Petrushevska Tozi, L., Mladenovska, K., Functional probiotic and synbiotic food products-advances in production, evaluation and health benefit. In: Injac, R. (Edit.). The Analysis of pharmacologically active compounds and biomolecules in real samples. Transworld Research Network, Kerala, India, p: 129-164 (2009).

Phillips M., Kailasapathy K., Tran L., Viability of commercial probiotic cultures (*L. acidophilus*, *Bifidobacterium* sp., *L. casei*, *L. paracasei*, and *L. rhamnosus*) in Cheddar cheese. Int. J. Food Microbiol. 108: 276-280 (2006).

Picot A., Lacroix C., Optimization of dynamic loop mixer operating conditions for production of o/w emulsion for cell microencapsulation. Le Lait 83: 237-250 (2003b).

Picot A., Lacroix C., Encapsulation of bifidobacteria in whey protein-based microcapsules and survival in simulated gastrointestinal conditions and in yoghurt. Int. Dairy J. 14(6): 505-515 (2004).

Ping S.U., Henriksson A., Mitchell H., Selected prebiotics support the growth of probiotic mono-cultures *in vitro*. Anaerobe 13: 134-139 (2007).

Pitkala K.H., Strandberg T.E., Finne-Soveri U.H., Ouwehand A.C., Poussa T., Salminen S., Fermented cereal with specific bifidobacteria normalizes bowel movements in elderly nursing home residents. A randomized controlled trial. J. Nutr. Health Aging 11(4): 305-311 (2007).

Pliszczak D., Bourgeois S., Bordes C., Valour J.P., Mazoyer M.A., Orecchioni A.M., Nakache E., Lantéri P., Improvement of an encapsulation process for the preparation of pro- and prebiotics-loaded bioadhesive microparticles by using experimental design. Eur. J. Pharm. Sci. 44: 83-92 (2011).

Prakash S., Tomaro-Duchesneau C., Saha S., Cantor A., The gut microbiota and human health: an emphasis on the use of microencapsulated bacterial cells. J. Biomed. Biotechnol. 2-12 (2011).

Rakin M., Vukasinovic M., Siler-Marinkovic S., Maksimovic M., Contribution of lactic acid fermentation to improved nutritive quality vegetable juices enriched with brewer's yeast autolysate. Food Chem. 100: 599-602 (2007).

Ranadheera R.D.C.S., Baines S.K., Adams M.C., Importance of food in probiotic efficacy. Food Res. Int. 43: 1-7 (2010).

Ray R.C., Sivakumar P.S., Traditional and novel fermented foods and beverages from tropical root and tuber crops: review. Int. J. Food Sci. Technol. 44(6): 1073-1087 (2009).

Roberfroid M.B., Global view on functional foods: European perspectives. Br. J. Nutr. 88: S133-S138 (2002).

Roberfroid M.B., Inulin-type fructans: Functional food ingredients. J. Nutr. 137: 2493S-2502S (2007b).

Rößle C., Brunton N., Gormley R.T., Ross P.R., Butler F., Development of potentially synbiotic fresh-cut apple slices. J. Funct. Foods 2: 245-254 (2010).

Roy C.C., Kien C.L., Bouthillier L., Levy E., Short-chain fatty acids: ready for prime time? Nutr. Clin. Pract. 21: 351-366 (2006).

Saad N., Delattre C., Urdaci M., Schmitter J.M., Bressollier P., An overview of the last advances in probiotic and prebiotic field. LWT-Food Sci. Technol. 50: 1-16 (2013).

Sánchez B., Ruiz L., Gueimonde M., Ruas-Madiedo P., Margolles A., Toward improving technological and functional properties of probiotics in foods. Trends Food Sci. Technol. 26: 56-63 (2012).

Sandoval-Castilla O., Lobato-Calleros C., Garcia-Galindo H.S., Alvarez-Ramirez J., Vernon-Carter E.J., Textural properties of alginate-pectin beads and survivability of entrapped *Lb. casei* in simulated gastrointestinal conditions and in yoghurt. Food Res. Int. 43: 111-117 (2010).

Sarkar S., Approaches for enhancing the viability of probiotics: a review. Br. Food J. 112(4): 329-349 (2010).

Schmitt J., Flemming H.C., FTIR-spectroscopy in microbial and material analysis. Int. Biodeter. Biodegr. 41: 1-11 (1998).

Shah N.P., Probiotic bacteria: Selective enumeration and survival in dairy foods. J. Dairy Sci. 83: 894-907 (2000).

Sheehan V.M., Ross P., Fitzgerald G.F., Assessing the acid tolerance and the technological robustness of probiotic cultures for fortification in fruit juices. Innov. Food Sci. Emerg. Technol. 8(2): 279-284 (2007).

Smilkov K., Petreska Ivanovska T., Petrushevska-Tozi L., Petkovska R., Hadjieva J., Popovski E., Stafilov T., Grozdanov A., Mladenovska K., Optimization of the formulation for the preparing of *Lactobacillus casei* loaded whey-protein-Ca-alginate microparticles using full-factorial design. J. Microencapsul. 31(2): 166-175 (2014).

Soccol C.R., de Souza Vandenberghe L.P., Spier, M.R., Medeiros A.B.P., Yamaguishi C.T., Lindner J.D.D., Pandey A., Thomaz-Soccol V., The potential of probiotics: a review. Food Technol. Biotecnol. 48(4): 413-434 (2010).

Sohail A., Turner M.S., Prabawati E.K., Coombes A.G.A., Bhandari B., Evaluation of *Lactobacillus rhamnosus* GG and *Lactobacillus acidophilus* NCFM encapsulated using a novel impinging aerosol method in fruit food products. Int. J. Food Microbiol. 157: 162-166 (2012).

Soukoulis C., Behboudi-Jobbehdar S., Yonekura L., Parmenter C., Stability of *Lactobacillus rhamnosus* GG in prebiotic edible films. Food Chem. 159: 302-308 (2014).

Talwalkar A., Kailasapathy K., A review of oxygen toxicity in probiotic yoghurts: influence on the survival of probiotic bacteria and protective techniques. Compreh. Rev. Food Sci. Food Safety 3(3): 117-124 (2004b).

Tamminen M., Salminen S., Ouwehand A.C., Fermentation of carrot juice by probiotics: viability and preservation of adhesion. Int. J. Biotechnol. Wellness Ind. 2: 10-15 (2013).

Tan J., McKenzie C., Potamitis M., Thornburn A.N., Mackay C.R., Macia L., The role of short-chain fatty acids in health and disease. Adv. Immunol. 121: 91-119 (2014).

Torres-Giner S., Martinez-Abad A., Ocio M.J., Lagaron M.J., Stabilization of a nutraceutical omega-3 fatty acid by encapsulation in utrathin electro-sprayed Zein Prolamine. J. Food Sci. 75(6): N69-N79 (2010).

Truelstrup Hansen L., Allan-Wojtas P.M., Jin Y.L., Paulson, A.T., Survival of Ca-alginate microencapsulated *Bifidobacterium spp.* in milk and simulated gastrointestinal conditions. Food Microbiol. 19: 35-45 (2002).

Tsen J.H., Lin Y.P., King V.A., Fermentation of banana media by using κ-carrageenan immobilized *Lactobacillus acidophilus*. Int. J. Food Microbiol. 91: 215-220 (2004).

Tsen J.H., Lin Y.P., Huang H.Y., King V.A., Studies on the fermentation of tomato juice by using κ-carrageenan immobilized *Lactobacillus acidophilus*. J. Food Process. Pres. 32: 178-189 (2008).

Vidhyalakshmi R., Bhakyaraj R., Subhasree R.S., Encapsulation "the future of probiotics"- a review. Adv. Biol. Res. 3: 96-103 (2009).

Vodnar D.C., Paucean A., Dulf F.V., Socaciu C., HPLC characterization of lactic acid formation and FTIR fingerprint of probiotic bacteria during fermentation processes. Not. Bot. Hort. Agrobot. Cluj 38: 109-113 (2010).

Vinderola G.C., Reinheimer J.A., Enumeration of *Lactobacillus casei* in the presence of *L. acidophilus*, Bifidobacteria and lactic starter bacteria in fermented dairy products. Int. Dairy J. 14(4): 271-275 (2000).

Ying D.Y., Phoon M.C., Sanguansri L., Weerakkody R., Burgar I., Augustin M.A., Microencapsulated *Lactobacillus rhamnosus* GG powders: relationship of powder physical properties to probiotic survival during storage. J. Food Sci. 75: 588-595 (2010).

Ying D., Schwander S., Weerakkody R., Sanguansri L., Gantenbein-Demarchi C., Augustin M., Microencapsulated *Lactobacillus rhamnosus* GG in whey protein and resistant starch matrices: probiotic survival in fruit juice. J. Funct. Foods 5(1): 98-105 (2012).

Wang Y.C., Yu R.C., Yang H.-Y., Chou C.C., Sugar and acid contents in soymilk fermented with lactic acid bacteria alone or simultaneously with bifidobacteria. Food Microbiol. 20: 333-338 (2003).

Washington N., Washington C., Wilson C.G., Physiological pharmaceutics – barriers to drug absorption. Taylor & Francis, London and New York, USA, p: 143-174 (2001).

Wickens K., Black P.N., Stanley T.V., A differential effect of 2 probiotics in the prevention of eczema and atopy: a doble-blined, randomized, placebo-controlled trial. J. Allergy Clin. Immunol. 122: 788-794 (2008).

Zhou Y., Martins E., Groboillot A., Champagne C.P., Neufeld R.J., Spectrophotometric quantification of lactic acid bacteria in alginate and control of cell release with chitosan coating. J. Appl. Microbiol. 84: 342-348 (1998).

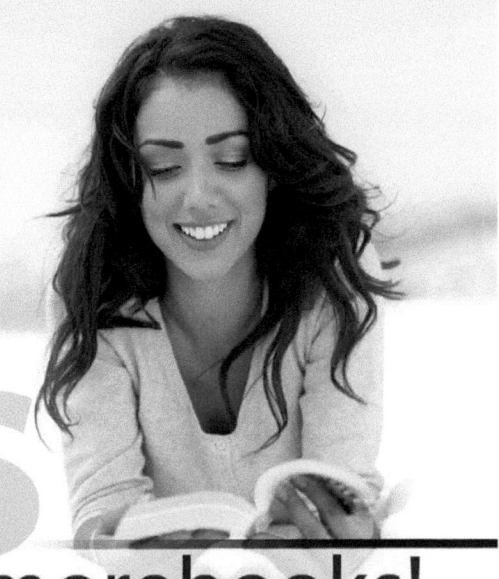
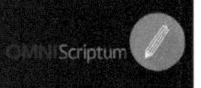

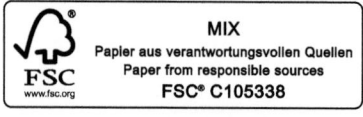